The Therapy
of
Natural Living

By Regina Nedas

Publisher's Page

Text and Photography by Regina Nedas
© Regina Nedas 2019

Published by
Doctor's Dreams Publishing
PO Box 4808
Biloxi, MS 39535

Prepared in the United States of America
Paperback edition printed in the USA by CreateSpace

ICBN: 978-1-942181-15-6
LCN:

Special thanks to Dr. Levin for his help in compiling and editing this book.

The Therapy of Natural Living

By Regina Nedas

Edited by Philip L. Levin, MD

Improve your health and vitality by recognizing the values of natural foods and health products.

Table of Contents

NOTE TO THE READER

Despite the emergence of an increasing number of new drugs and the expansion of their production and use, one should not forget that our ancestors successfully used natural medicinal plants for their health needs. This "folk medicine" still works, and this book provides a guide to those plants and their uses.

This book is not meant to offer medical advice or prescriptions, and one should be cautious not to risk self-diagnosis. We recommend only using herbal medicines after a proper consultation from a qualified herbalist and/or physician. Remember, while many specialists can help you with your health, a state-licensed medical doctor should be consulted to confirm any medical condition. Some herbal medicines might interact with prescribed medications. If unexpected symptoms occur after trying herbal remedies, stop taking the treatments and consult a competent professional. Always use medicinal plants with care and discretion; they are, after all medicines.

ADVICE ABOUT COLLECTING PLANTS

The best locations for harvesting medicinal plants are mountain peaks and forests where the soil is rich in minerals and air is extremely clean. For those plants that grow in fields and grasslands, try to find areas where people rarely enter. These plants have the advantage of untainted therapeutic properties. Because plants intensively store poisonous substances they find in their environment, try to avoid collecting medicinal plants growing on roadsides, or in the fields near industrial plants, large cities, railways, motorways, or in other obviously contaminated areas.

Because most of the active substances are present in the upper part of the herbaceous stem, the best time to harvest medicinal plants is before flowering or at the beginning of flowering.

Dry your plants in shaded, warm, well-ventilated rooms and then store them in tightly-closed jars, clay pots, wooden containers, or paper bags in dry rooms. Leaves, flowers, herbs, and non-temperate fruits of juvenile plants should not be collected after rain or during the early morning when they still are covered with dew because they will not dry as well.

As many plants look alike, be sure you can properly identify the plants you pick yourself. If in doubt, show them to a trusted herbalist before using them.

PREFACE

Hippocrates said: "Food is your medicine, and medicine is your food." This saying is as relevant today as it was two thousand years ago.

I lived in Europe for many years and taught botany and microbiology in an agricultural college. Here I developed my interest in medical plants, their harvesting, and their applications in folk medicine. Many plants and chemicals in nature have healing benefits on the human body. Over the years, I've studied folk medicine literature, collecting recommendations from around the world about healthy lifestyles, ethnic medicine, and natural curative techniques.

In this age of modern pharmaceuticals, homeopathic treatments have lost adherents. Yet I know from my studies how useful this knowledge can be. The day will come again when people realize the great values of ethnic herbal remedies and natural treatment methods.

I acquired knowledge of ethnic medicine in my travels through Lithuania, Russia, The Caucasus, India, Pakistan, and North America. From each area I interviewed natives and studied old texts to acquire information about medicinal herbal treatments, much of it unique and ancient. I have collected this information and integrated it with modern scientific knowledge to present the best applications of medicinal plants in folk medicine. I want to share this information with all the readers who are interested in the natural world.

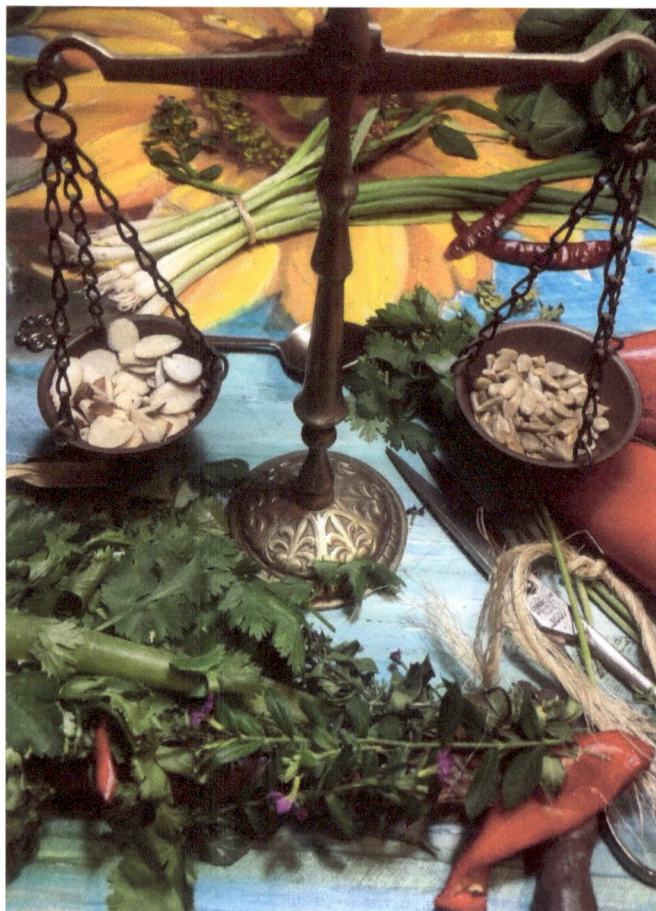

INTRODUCTION

"Away from the tumult of motor and mill. I want to be carefree,
I want to be still!
I'm weary of doing things; weary of words
I want to be one with the blossoms and birds."
– Edgar A. Guest, 1881-1959.

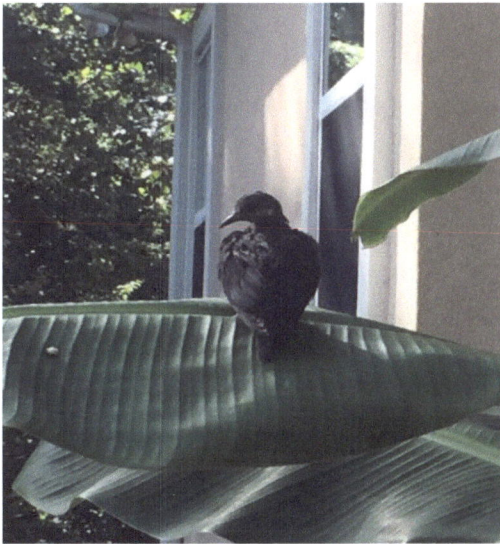

While living in the age of technology with the current pace of modern life, we have forgotten from where we came. Penetrating the pleasures of civilization makes it easy to relinquish the innate connection with nature, which has been, first and foremost, a source of joy for adults and children alike. Old mythology, religion, and related rituals are phenomena of spiritual creativity, all of which have helped to draw from the forces of nature, look for harmony in nature, and teach how to improve health by natural means. We need to understand our natural environment around us, stretch out our hands, and work with it together. Only then will we achieve the radiant strength from nature that will allow us to properly choose ingredients botanical gardens provide, in the same vein as true natural healers.

In the past, the basis of human life was in finding harmony with nature by observing its laws. It is only when humans found harmony with nature that they were able to adapt to it. In achieving this, humans thrived. By following nature's guides, we can cherish nature's miracles. Fusion with nature improves an individual's psychology and physiology and reduces stress.

INVITING NATURE INTO OUR LIVES

I arise today
Through the strength of heaven:
Light of Sun,
Radiance of Moon,
Splendor of fire,
Speed of lightning,
Swiftness of wind,
Depth of sea,
Stability of Earth,
Firmness of rock.
– Saint Patrick, 385 - 461 AD

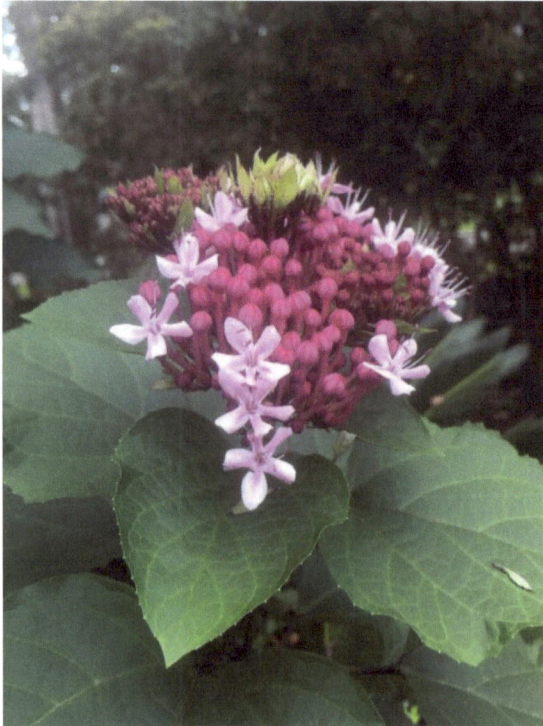

Nature is fascinating yet unfamiliar, but it also inspires us every step of the way; consequently, nature changes constantly, thus providing us with plenty of happy moments. Every time we see nature, it is different. Meadows play host to verdant and flourishing plants with different flavors at different times. Let us feel the scents of the forest, of flowers in bloom, freshly cut grass, and the bitterness of the pine needles. These colorful mosaics instill delight in every one of us. Natural garden scents conjure feelings of mysticism, massaging both the body and soul, allowing us to get acquainted with nature and its wealth and learning how to make tools that enhance beauty and maintain health. In doing this, we can find true harmony with nature.

"No man can taste the fruits of autumn while he is delighting this scent with the flowers of spring."

– Samuel Johnson, 1709-1784.

The soul of the human being enjoys music, poetry, and theater. This is wonderful, but our soul also needs to feel the beauty of nature and inhale its fragrant air. Nature is so important to us. It doesn't matter if we live in the countryside or in the city, since each scent of flowers, grass, and trees delights us, allowing us to feel free from stress and bad thoughts and increasing good emotions.

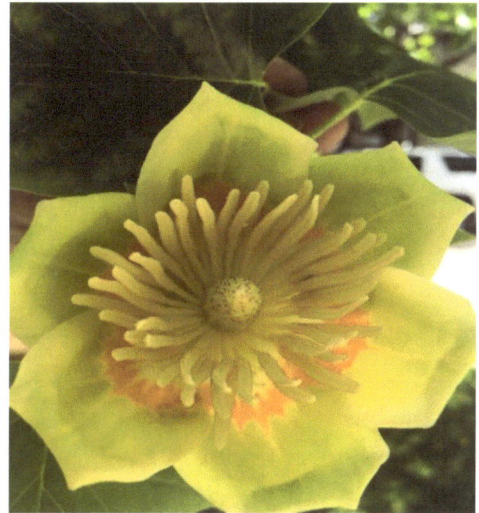

ANIMALS KNOW HOW TO HEAL THEMSELVES

It is not only humans that seek out drugs to relieve a stomach ache, get rid of a headache, or treat a skin condition—animals do this too. By instinct, animals know how to heal themselves if they feel sick by using the natural healing forces of nature. Growing scientific evidence indicates that animals have an innate knowledge of natural medicine. In fact, they have access to the world's largest pharmacy: nature itself.

Zoologists and botanists are only just beginning to understand how animals use plants to prevent and cure illness, specifically how animals use seeds, leaves, roots, and barks as well as minerals to treat a variety of ailments. Many folk remedies have come from noticing which plants animals eat when they are sick. Dogs and cats naturally cure their stomach upsets by eating grass and making themselves vomit. Horses have a well-developed sense of taste and are very picky in choosing their food. For example, they never eat smelly oats or poisonous plants, and they do not drink smelly water. In the springtime they eat fresh dandelions to purify their blood.

An important discovery was once made when a pregnant African elephant was observed for over a year. The elephant set off in search for a shrub that grew 17 miles from her usual food source. The elephant chewed the leaves and bark of the bush, only to give birth a few days later. This plant is a member of the Borage family and is brewed by Kenyan women to make a labor-inducing tea. In addition, chimps eat the Aspilia shrub, which produces bristly leaves. They peel the stems and eat the pith of the Vernonia plant. This plant was found to have antiparasitic and antimicrobial properties. Both Aspilia and Vernonia plants have long been used in Tanzanian folk medicine for stomach upsets and fever.

Many animals eat minerals such as clay or charcoal for their curative properties. Colobus monkeys on the island of Zanzibar have been observed stealing and eating charcoal from human bonfires. The charcoal counteracts the toxic phenols produced by the mango and almond leaves which make up their diet. South American parrots and macaws are known to eat soil with a high kaolin content. The parrots' diet contains toxins because of the fruit seeds they eat. The kaolin clay absorbs the toxins and carries them out of the birds' digestive systems, thus leaving the parrots unharmed by the poisons. Kaolin has been used in many cultures as a remedy for human gastrointestinal problems.

NATURE PROTECTS US—NATURE TREATS US—
NATURE IS A BIG PHARMACY

Medicus-Curat, Natura-sanat. Medicine protects, nature heals.
– St. Hildegard von Bingen, 1098-1179. CAUSAE ET CURAE.

"The Lord has created medicines out of the earth; and he that is wise will not abhor them"
– King James Version, Ecclesiasticus 38:4

In ancient times, people harnessed the power of healing herbs, plants, fruits, and oils to take care of their health, life expectancy, strength, endurance, working capacity, ability to work, and their energy levels. During these times, prophets also proposed treatments with medicinal plant concoctions and extracts against diseases and disabilities. The nobility studied phytotherapy ("herbal treatment") at the European Universities, in multiple languages, learning of medical therapies from many cultures.

Frequently, the library of the aristocrat contained the *Canon of Medicine*, written by Persian physician Avicenna (980-1037). Nowadays, many professors teach from this book at European Universities. Avicenna is regarded as one of the most significant physicians of the Islamic Golden Age and was described as the father of early modern medicine. His short name was Ibn Sina. Another classic herbalist text is St. Hildegard von Bingen's *Causae et Curae*. These healers gathered information from early cultures across the known world, including Greece, Rome, Babylon, Egypt, China, Tibet, and India. In India the method was called Ayurveda, a format that continues to be popular today.

Egyptians took their health very seriously, claiming to be the healthiest people in the world after the Libyans. They practiced the ritual of cleanliness. Because soap was still unknown, they used ashes or soda which are both good detergents and dissolve fatty matter. Both men and woman removed hair from their entire bodies and anointed their heads with scented oils. Those who wished to erase the marks of the years and to prevent the appearance of wrinkles, freckles, and other outrages of age used extracted fenugreek oil. Body smell had always been a matter of concern in the civilized East where prescriptions for perfumes were profuse.

Amenemhat III (1840-1792 B.C.) propagated the Kahn Papyrus which dates from 1950 B.C. It consists of three sections, one dealing with human medicine, the second with veterinary science, and the third with mathematics. Its first two pages contains seventeen gynecological prescriptions and instructions. Substances recommended are beer, milk, oil, dates, and herbs.

The Ramesseum IV and V papyri were probably written about 1900 B.C., about the same epoch as the Kahn Papyrus. Papyrus IV is very similar to the Kahn Papyrus, while papyrus V is purely medical. This papyrus was written in hieroglyphic script and contains twenty prescriptions of which many are dealing with relaxing "stiffened" limbs.

The Ebers Papyrus is the longest of all the known papyri and the most important, considering the physiological and medicinal knowledge. It comes from the 9th year of the reign of Amenophis I (1550 B.C.). The sections contain information on digestion and worms and their treatment, sections on eye diseases, on the care of the skin, hair and other issues.

The descriptions are pretty often poetic. A weak person is compared to a "breath that passes away." Many are remarkable in their prescriptions for problems such as those for angina pectoris, aneurysm, and hernia.

Hippocrates treatment methods

- First of all do not hurt (primum non nocere).
- Make full use of nature (Natura senat, medicus curat).
- Contrary (contraris curantur).

The Medical Literature of Antiquity. The oldest doctor of early medical history is considered to be the Greek physician, philosopher Hippocrates of Cos (460-370 B.C.), to whom modern doctors give a professional oath. Hippocrates originated from the tribes of the Ascension, who associated their skills from the healing god of Asclepius. Hippocrates, is considered to be the father of today's medicine. He believed in the healing power of nature and medical observation. The diagnostic system introduced by Hippocrates was based on a logical interpretation of illnesses rather than the prevailing belief of the "will of the gods." Using healing plants and herbs, he developed his famous theory of four types of body fluids and causes of illness. According to these liquids, he distinguished four of human temperaments - sangvinic, phlegmatic, choleric and melancholic, and the four elements acting on them: heat, cold, humidity and dryness, which must be in order to restore balance.

Of all his written work, only the "Corpus Hippocraticum" has been preserved, where the work of several writers called Hippocrates was assembled. From this we can list several medicinal herbs used by Hippocrates: rosemary, thyme, mint, fennel, cumin, rose, cloves, incense, mira (aromatic spices), calendula, garlic, scallop, and mandragora.

One of the greatest ancient Roman doctors was the Greek Asclepius (in Greek mythology, Asclepius is the god of medicine and healing), who came from Asia Minor. He was the first Greek medical practitioner to gain the confidence of the Romans. Asclepius prescribed only ordinary, natural substances to his patients. He prescribed wine as a medicine, either cold or hot and with salt or pepper. His main treatment method was to be "fast and pleasant" (cito, tuto et jucunde). The Asclepios cult systematized the knowledge of the Ayurveda, Chinese, Persian, Greek, Roman, and Tibetan systems and used the traditional medical system to develop diagnostic methods that allowed the individual to choose an appropriate treatment. They used plant extracts for treatment, producing many of these compounds themselves, and recommended treatments from plants growing in the same place where a sick person was. With these influences, over the centuries plants and people have adapted to each other.

In ancient times, some of the most effective drugs were composited from what was called six berry wine: raspberries, blueberries, blackcurrant, redcurrant, cranberries, and cherries. There was also a famous dandelion wine used prominently in Europe.

Across the world and throughout history, folk herbalists have used the medicines and remedies found in the largest pharmacy on earth: nature itself.

WHAT WE LEARN FROM OUR DISEASES

"It would not be good if all our desires were fulfilled: only when we become ill, we understand what kind of wealth is health, only having experienced evil, we appreciate the goodness, only when we are hungry, we feel the taste of meal, only when we get tired, we are enjoying the rest".
–Heraclitus, Greek philosopher, 535 BC-475 BC.

In order to stay healthy or to recover faster from illnesses, it is important to bear a few things in mind; namely, to enjoy every moment of our lives, love yourself and others sincerely, laugh, and have as much fun as possible. It is important to learn from our experiences and to get rid of erratic stereotypes.

CHAPTER 1

HONEY AND CINNAMON

"Honey is the flower transmuted – its scent and beauty transformed into aroma and taste."
— Stephanie Rosenbaum, food writer.

The famous Persian physician Avicenna once advised: "If you want to stay young, be sure to eat honey."

Ayurvedic doctors, as well as those practicing Yunani medicine, have used honey as a medicine for centuries. Modern scientists recognize honey as an extremely effective medication that treats many illnesses.

Honey is absorbed quickly, and the burst of glucose rapidly restores human energy levels. In addition to honey's delicious taste, it also has huge benefits for the human body with its antioxidants and antiviral, antimicrobial, and antifungal properties.

One tablespoon of honey contains 64 calories. The composition of honey is as follows: 80% carbohydrates, 18% water, and 2% vitamins and minerals. Honey does not contain any fat, cholesterol, or amino acids. It is a sweetener, with its main ingredients being glucose and fructose.

Honey is particularly useful for long term storage because if kept properly, it won't spoil. When stored for long periods, honey can crystallize, though crystallization does not change its properties; it will never degenerate to its sugars. To turn the crystals back to liquid, place the jar in a warm water bath. The bath should not be too hot because high temperatures destroy some of the honey's antibacterial action. Honey should never be heated above 37°C (98.6°F), for at that temperature some of the protective enzymes break down. For the same reason, store your honey away from direct sunlight.

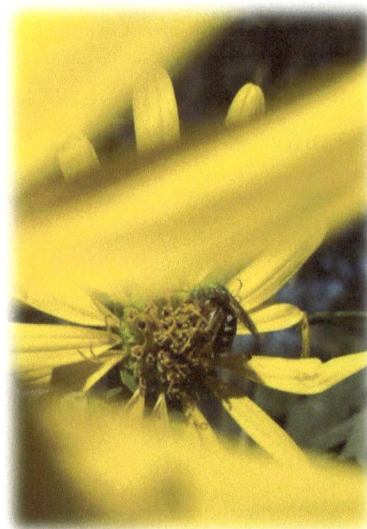

In winter time if you buy the liquid form of honey and find that it won't crystallize, that might be because the honey has been heated above 40 C (104 F). Sometimes the seller will heat honey to stop the process of fermentation that may have already begun. The nutritional and healing values of overheated honey are greatly reduced.

HOW TO DISTINGUISH NATURAL FROM ARTIFICAL HONEY

First read the labels on the product. If the honey contains some impurities, the label must indicate the percentage of honey contained in the product;

Rub a small amount of honey between your fingers, warm honey gently penetrates into the skin and is not as sticky as honey with additives or artificial honey;

Put a small drop of honey on a newspaper. Liquid natural honey will bead up because it only contains a very small amount of water, while artificial honey will create a wet halo, due to higher water content.

Add a teaspoon of honey to an egg yolk and beat with a fork. Real honey will mix with the yolk to create a smooth blend. Artificial or sugar syrup will not blend.

Put a teaspoon of honey in a glass with water. Natural honey will cover the bottom of the glass while artificial or sugar syrup will dissolve.

When natural honey is spread on a slice of bread, it hardens quickly. Artificial honey will make the bread surface moist due to its increased amount of water.

Natural honey creates a tingling sensation in the throat; artificial does not cause such a feeling; it will simply be drunk as a simple sugar solution.

Over time, natural honey eventually crystallizes while artificial honey always looks like a sugar solution.

Place a sample of your honey onto a toothpick and hold a flame under it. Natural honey will burn, and artificial honey (due to higher water content) will not.

Heating 2-3 teaspoons of honey in a microwave oven will cause it to quickly caramelizes without bubbles (such as boiling water) while heated honey with impurities or sugar syrup produces bubbles and the product will not caramelize.

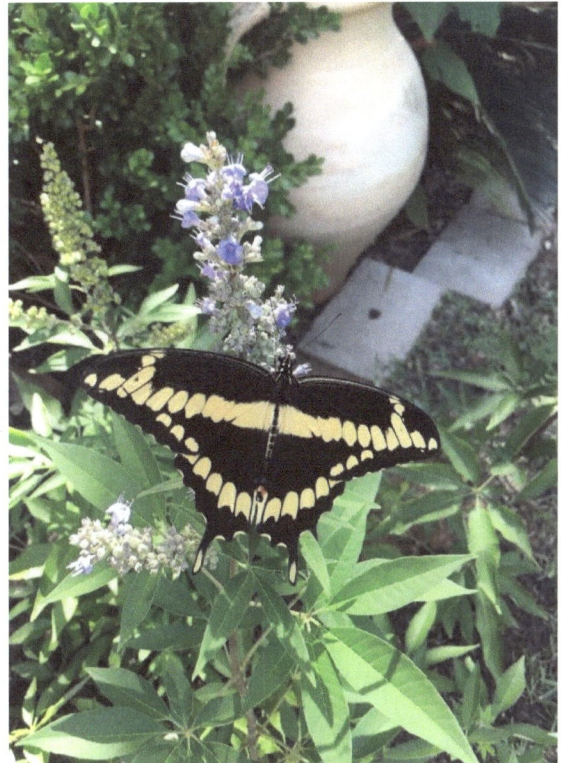

THE HEALTH BENEFITS OF HONEY

Honey acts as a calming agent, thus it is particularly beneficial for nervous, hard-working people and those with poor sleeping habits. Honey strengthens the immune system and prevents anemia. Many people find it to be an excellent remedy for cough. When chewing honey with honeycombs, there is a prophylactic effect of the respiratory tract.

The recommended dose for protection of the immune system is one teaspoon daily.

Children under one year of age should not be given honey due to their susceptibility to botulism. If honey is accidentally inhaled, it damages the bronchial tree, so it should be used cautiously in those with lung diseases. Due to its sugar content, diabetics and overweight people must be careful with its use, and, of course, those allergic to honey shouldn't consume it.

Yunani and Ayurvedic medicine have traditionally used honey as a means of enhancing the sperm. In addition, regularly ingesting 2 tablespoons of honey before bedtime has been said to cure impotence.

Yunani Medicine

Yunani medicine is the traditional medicine practiced in parts of India and in some Muslim cultures in South and Central Asia. The term "Yunani" means "Greek" in Arabic, for its roots are based on the technics of the Greek physicians Hippocrates and Galen. Formalized in the eleventh century "The Canon of Medicine," it spread through India and the Mughal Empire during the 13th century.

INTERESTING FACTS ABOUT HONEY

- In ancient Egypt, honey was used for embalming the dead.
- The Arabs have traditionally used honey as a preservative for meat.
- The ancient Vikings used honey and bee bread for going on long journeys – one tablespoon helped to restore their energy levels.
- The ancient Greeks believed that honey could prolong life. They explained their gods' immortality and eternal youthfulness by the fact that they ate ambrosia—a mixture of honey and milk.
- The ancient Roman poet Ovidius, in his works about the golden age, claimed that this period was famous for dairy and nectar rivers and honey dropping from the green oak.
- Honey is a mandatory food included in an astronaut's diet.
- Beekeepers say that the best honey is found in the honeycombs as it retains all the healing properties. Our ancestors ate honey with honeycombs, as well as bee bread.

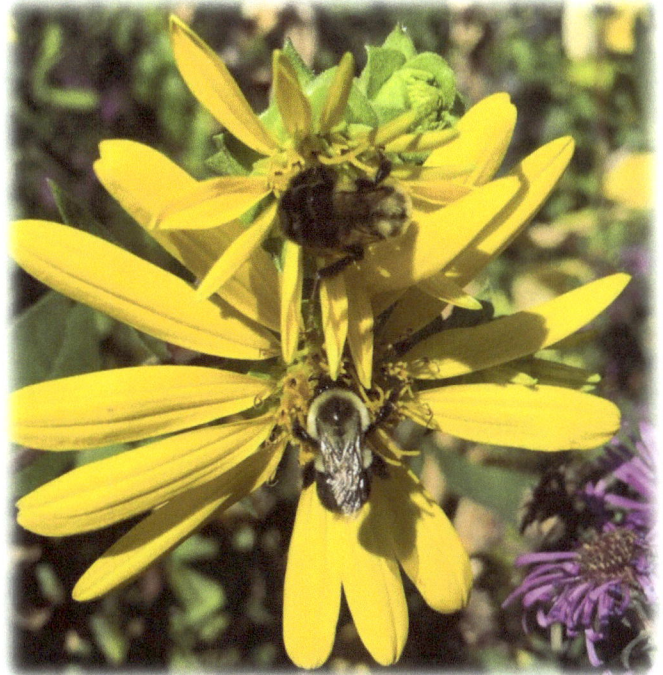

CINNAMON

Cinnamon has been used by humans for thousands of years, noted by its mention in the Old Testament for its benefits as an anointing and perfuming oil. Throughout history it's been valued, a prime item on the Spice Trail from Asia into Europe during the Middle Ages.

The four basic commercially available types are Ceylon Cinnamon, Cassia or Chinese Cinnamon, Saigon Cinnamon, and Korintje Cinnamon. Chinese cinnamon, mostly produced in Indonesia, is the primary cinnamon found in North America, and Ceylon cinnamon, produced in Sri Lanka, the most widely used in Europe. The purest form with the strongest healing ingredients is the Ceylon cinnamon (Cinnamomum zeylanicium). I prefer this brand over the cassia types produced in Indonesia, China, and Vietnam, easily distinguished as the cassia is muddy brown while the color of genuine cinnamon is light brown. If you buy cinnamon sticks, you'll find that cassia sticks are very hard and are tucked in the form of a hollow tube. Because of their density, they're especially difficult to grind. Genuine Ceylon cinnamon sticks are thin and brittle and easily broken, and the inside has a full-bodied, cigarette-like appearance. See the photo that demonstrates the difference.

When sold in a store, cinnamon might be a mixture of many products, sometimes with so little actual cinnamon it seems like colored and scented sawdust. The most reliable way to buy cinnamon is from specialized spice shops, or to buy cinnamon sticks and grind them yourself into a powder.

The benefits of cinnamon are numerous. For example, it is a strong antioxidant and protects the body from cancer, heart disease, inflammation, and premature aging. Half a teaspoon a day can reduce the amount of bad cholesterol in the blood and may help to treat type 2 diabetes as it reduces the amount of sugar in the blood, increases insulin production, and aids weight loss. Cinnamon has an antibacterial effect. Some studies suggest it can slow down the cancer cell growth of leukemia and lymphoma and reduce the risk of blood clots. Cinnamon is also a perfect natural preservative. Smelling cinnamon can improve the blood circulation in the brain. Be sure you use genuine cinnamon, as some cassia has been reported to cause liver damage. Cinnamon should be taken in moderation, with one teaspoon the daily recommended

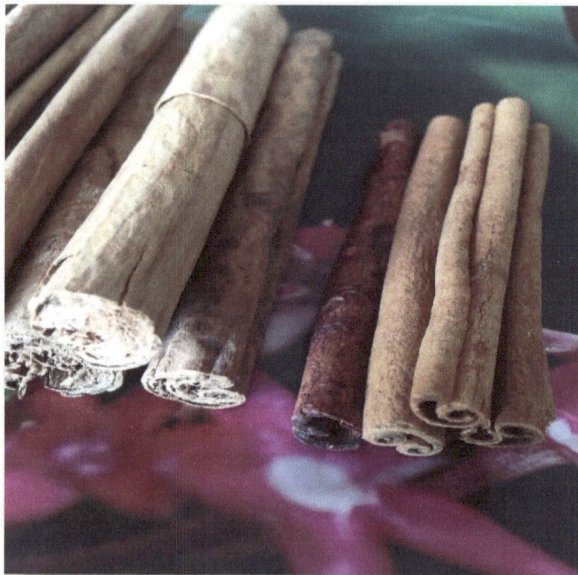

amount. Tea, coffee, and various desserts can be flavored with this spice. Since ancient times in China, Japan, and other parts of the Far East, women who have been unable to get pregnant or wanted to strengthen their womb have used cinnamon powder.

.

BENEFITS OF COMBINING HONEY AND CINNAMON

Canadian Magazine "Weekly World News" date 01/17/1995 published a list of diseases that can be treated with honey and cinnamon (as proven by modern medical research). When applying honey and cinnamon as a treatment, it is necessary to cut out or at least reduce the use of sugar.

1. Heart disease: Use honey and cinnamon mash and put it on a slice of bread instead of using preserves and jam. If you eat this kind of slice for breakfast daily, it will reduce cholesterol levels and protect against heart attacks. If you have already suffered from a heart attack, this mash will protect against recurrences. These breakfasts also restore the elasticity of the artery and vein walls and improve the blood vessel condition. Many elderly rest-homes have used this honey and cinnamon mash in Canada and America for years.

2. Arthritis: People with arthritis should drink a cup of hot water with 2 teaspoons of honey and 1 teaspoon of cinnamon in the morning and in the evening. Even chronic arthritis is improved if you drink regularly. The University of Copenhagen conducted a study in which patients ate 1 teaspoon of honey with half a teaspoon of cinnamon each morning before breakfast. Out of 200 subjects, 73 patients stated that their pain had disappeared within one month.

3. Bladder infections: Mix 1 teaspoon of cinnamon with 1 teaspoon of honey in a warm cup of water. This concoction can clear bacteria from the urinary bladder.

4. Colds: Ingesting 1 teaspoon of honey with half a teaspoon of cinnamon three times a day helps clear the sinus congestion symptoms associated with colds, such as coughs and stuffy noses.

5. Stomach, digestive disorders, gas: Indian and Japanese scientists have noticed that honey mixed with cinnamon can treat digestive disorders. Sprinkling cinnamon powder on two tablespoons of honey and consuming before eating helps to digest even the heaviest of foods and reduces the accumulation of gas in the intestine.

6 Immune system: The daily use of honey and cinnamon strengthens immunity and protects the body against viruses and bacteria. Honey contains plenty of vitamins, minerals, and iron, all of which strengthen the white blood cells.

7. Heartburn: It is recommended to eat two teaspoons of honey sprinkled with cinnamon before meals. This mixture reduces acidity and improves digestion.

8. Sore throat: Add a tablespoon of honey to a cup of hot milk. Drink the milk slowly with the melted honey. Repeat this procedure every 3 hours until the sore throat is gone.

9. Acne and other skin conditions: 3 tablespoons of honey and 1 teaspoon of cinnamon will help to reduce or even cure acne. Rub a thin layer of this mash over areas affected with acne before bedtime and wash it with warm water in the morning. This mash may help eczema and other rashes as well.

10. Losing weight: In the morning, half an hour before meals, and before going to bed, drink a cup of hot tea with cinnamon and honey on an empty stomach. This pre-prandial dose will reduce your appetite and promote weight loss.

11. Cholesterol: Mixing 2 tablespoons of honey and 1/3 teaspoon of cinnamon into 500 ml water will reduce the amount of cholesterol in the blood by up to 10%. The recommend dosage for this mixture is three times a day.

12. Longevity: Drinking tea with honey and cinnamon regularly can reduce signs of aging and prolong life. To do this, add 4 tablespoons of honey, 1 tablespoon of cinnamon, and 3 cups of water to a teapot and make a tea. Drink 1/4 cup 3 times a day.

13. Cancer: Studies conducted in Japan and Australia showed that people with advanced bowel and bone cancer benefitted from consuming a tablespoon of honey mixed with a teaspoon of cinnamon three times a day.

14. Fatigue: Older people who regularly use honey and cinnamon in equal parts are more vivacious and more flexible. A Dr. Milton recommended ½ a tablespoon each of honey and cinnamon in a glass of water in the morning and at 3 p.m. when the vitality of the body begins to decrease. An increase in vitality should be noted within a week of using this regimen.

15. Halitosis: South American people rinse their mouths and throats with a mixture of one teaspoon of honey and cinnamon in a glass of hot water in the morning. This helps to get rid of bad smells in the mouth during the day.

16. Deterioration of hearing: Regular use of honey and cinnamon may prevent further hearing loss and even improve hearing.

17. Hair Loss: A home-made paste may prevent further hair loss, and even restore some that has been lost, by stimulating hair follicles. Make a paste of hot olive oil mixed with 1 tablespoon of honey and 1 teaspoon of cinnamon powder. After cooling, use the paste on the head before washing, letting it soak for about 15 minutes, and then wash your head as usual.

18. Support of brain protective functions: According to conducted studies, the antioxidants present in cinnamon can help to protect the brain from oxidative damage and make the cells resistant to damage and mutation. These properties can help prevent Parkinson's disease, Alzheimer's disease, and similar age-related disorders.

19. Fertility: Old folk medicine books state that women who cannot get pregnant can mix a little cinnamon powder with half a teaspoon of honey. This mixture should be applied as often as possible to the gums several times a day. In doing this, the drug slowly mixes with saliva and it is absorbed into the body.

RECIPE:

Oranges with Honey and Cinnamon

Ingredients:
¼ cup of honey
1 teaspoon of grounded cinnamon
5 peeled oranges cut across into slices

Preparation:
1. Mix honey and cinnamon in a medium-sized glass jar.
2. Gently blend in the oranges until they are covered with honey.
3. Leave for 15 minutes before serving.

The effect of the orange is cooling, so the cinnamon's heat provides a balance. This dish greatly improves digestion and helps to restore body fluids. Many Chinese doctors use this formula to treat eye problems.

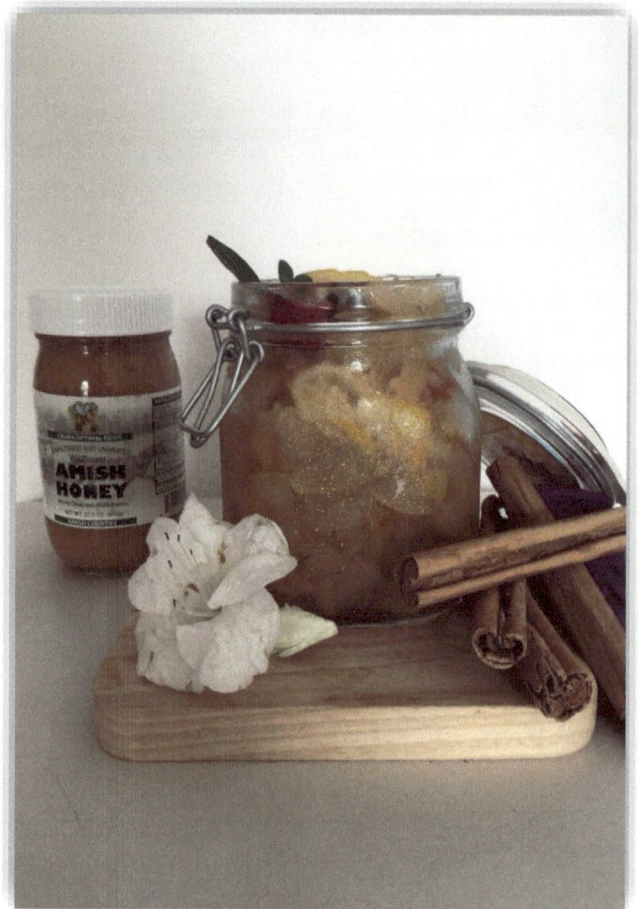

CHAPTER 2

SPICE

And God said, "Behold, I have given you every herb bearing seed, which is upon the face of all the earth, and every tree, in the which is the fruit of a tree yielding seed; to you it shall be meat."
– Holy Bible (King James Version).

The secret to happiness is variety, but the secret of variety, like the secret of all spices, is knowing when to use it.
— Daniel Gilbert, writer and psychologist.

What is a spice: A spice is a seed, fruit root, bark, or other plant substance, as compared to an herb, which is the leaf, flower, or stem. Either one may be used for flavoring, coloring, or preservation. Harmonizing spices in food is a great art. Many have a sharp taste and smell, so only a very small amount of spice will make a significant difference to the taste of the food you are preparing.

Botanical basis
- Seeds, such as fennel, mustard, nutmeg, and black pepper;
- Fruits, such as cayenne pepper, arils, and mace (part of the nutmeg plant);
- Barks, such as cinnamon and cassia;
- Flower buds, such as cloves;
- Stigmas, such as saffron;
- Roots, such as turmeric, ginger, and galangal;
- Resins, such as asafoetida.

Spices contain many biologically active substances. Each plant has an effect and therefore it is important to know their properties well before use. For example, paprika can be used to reduce atherosclerosis.

The most commonly used spices and herbs in culinary are listed below:

Allspice (Pimenta dioica)
Asafoetida (Ferula assafoetida)
Basil (Laurus nobilis)
Caraway (Carum carvi)
Cardamom (Elettaria cardamomum)
Cassia (Cinnamomum aromatic)
Cayenne pepper (Capsicum frutescens)
Celery leaf (Apium graveolens)
Chili pepper (Capsicum spp.)
Chives (Allium schoenoprasum)
Chervil (Anthriscus cerefolium)
Cilantro (Coriandrum sativum)
Cinnamon true or Ceylon (Cinnamomum verum)
Clove (Syzygium aromaticum)
Coriander seeds (Coriandrum sativum)
Cumin (Cuminum cyminum)
Curry leaf (Murraya koenigii)
Dill herb (Anethum graveolens)
Dill seed (Anethum graveolens)
Fennel (Foeniculum vulgare)
Galingale (Cyperus spp.)
Garlic chives (Allium tuberosum)
Ginger (Zingiber officinale)
Horseradish (Armoracia rusticana)
Lavender (Lavandula spp.)
Lemon balm (Melissa officinalis)
Marjoram (Origanum majorana)
Mint (Mentha spp.)
Mustard yellow (Brassica hirta=Sinapis alba)
Nutmeg (Myristica fragrans)
Oregano (Origanum vulgare)
Paprika (Capsicum annuum)
Parsley (Petroselinum crispum)
Pepper (black, white, or green) (Piper nigrum)
Peppermint (Mentha piperita)
Rosemary (Rosmarinus officinalis)
Safflower (Carthamus tinctorius)
Sage (Salvia officinalis)
Tarragon (Artemisia dracunculus)
Thyme (Thymus vulgaris
Turmeric (Curcuma longa)
Vanilla (Vanilla planifolia)

SPACE FOR NOTES:

THE HISTORY OF SPICES

The spice trade developed throughout South Asia and the Middle East at least 2000 BCE with cinnamon and black pepper, while East Asia mainly traded herbs and pepper. The Egyptians traditionally used herbs for mummification, and their demand for exotic spices and herbs helped stimulate world trade. The word spice comes from the Latin root word *spec*, a noun referring to "appearance, sort, or kind." It evolved in Old French into *espice*, which later became *epice.* By 1000 BCE, medical systems based upon herbs could be found in China, Korea, and India. Early uses were connected with magic, medicine, religion, and preservation.

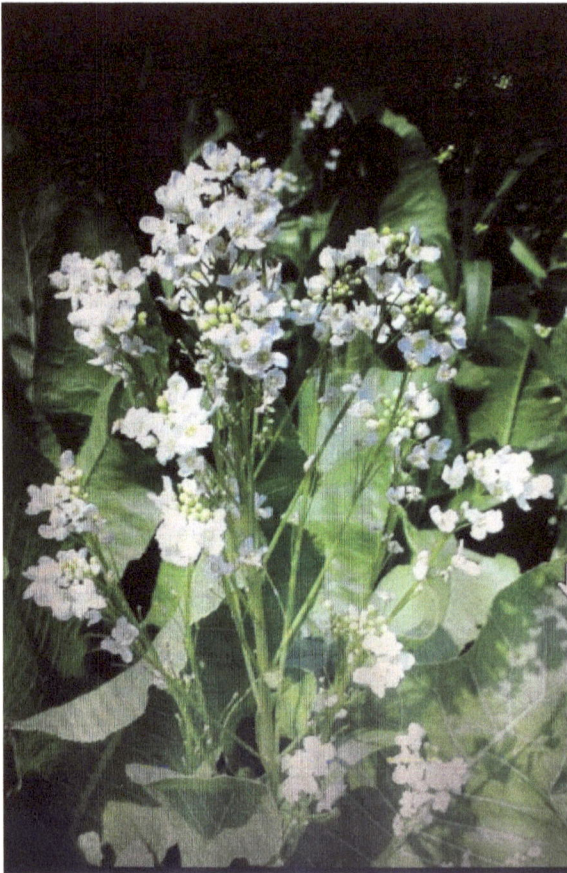

Spices were among the most demanded and expensive products available in Europe and in the Middle Ages, especially black pepper, cinnamon (and the cheaper alternative cassia), cumin, nutmeg, ginger, and cloves. Medieval medicine's main theory of the importance of balancing of the body's internal humors emphasized the use of spices and herbs. The European aristocracies demanded spices for both health and for the flavoring they added to their otherwise bland diets. The 12th century Spanish King of Aragon, for example, invested substantial resources into obtaining spices for his wine production.

Other information about Spices: Spices have a number of therapeutic properties. Many spices have antimicrobial properties, such as cumin, fresh ginger, and paprika. Paprika contains about 1122 IU of Vitamin A, while sea cabbage contains a lot of iodine. When it is missing, the lack of iodine affects the thyroid gland and healthy brain function. Spices are often used in medicine, religious rituals, cosmetics, perfume production, or as a vegetable. Spices are typically stored in sealed glass or metal containers in a dark closet.

Ginger

About Ginger (Zingiber officinale). Ginger is in the family Zingiberaceae. It is a herbaceous perennial that grows around stems about a meter tall bearing narrow green leaves and yellow flowers. Both the spicy leaves and the ginger root have been used as a natural medicine for more than 2000 years. Most of the ginger we use comes from China.

Ginger Health Benefits

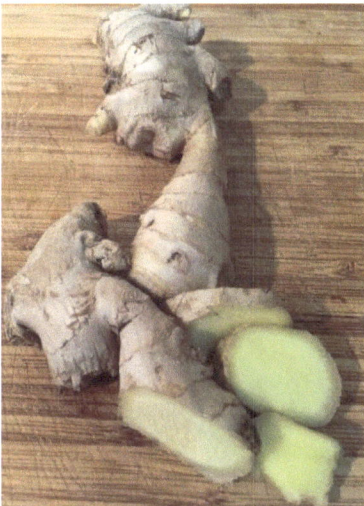

1. Heart Protection. It reduces blood clotting and can serve as a preventive measure against stroke and heart attacks.

2. Aid for Digestion. It helps to relieve constipation. In the morning, put a slice of cut ginger in a cup of boiled water, cover the cup, leave for 10-15 minutes (until the ginger is absorbed) and drink.

3. Flu Prevention. Add some sliced ginger to a cup of boiled water. After allowing the mixture to cool, add pressed lemon juice and a teaspoon of honey.

4. Immunity Enhancement. Ayurvedic medicine recommends using ginger as a spice to strengthen the immune system.

5. Prevention of cancer. As an antioxidant, ginger fights against aggressive and severe forms of lung, colon, breast, prostate, and ovarian cancer.

6. Prevention of diabetes. Studies have shown that ginger can contribute to healing diabetes. Ginger reduces the sugar content in the blood, as well as excess fat and cholesterol.

7. Menstrual pains. Ginger can help young women suffering from menstrual pains.

Warnings about the use of ginger: It can interact with many medications, such as anti-inflammatory drugs, heart pills, and blood thinners. Ginger can cause allergies during pregnancy, and worsen certain illnesses, such as gallbladder stones, stomach ulcers, herpes, and acne. Ginger suppresses the absorption of iron and fat-soluble vitamins. Due to blood thinning effects, it shouldn't be used within two weeks of anticipated surgery.

USING GINGER IN FOOD

Fresh ginger is commonly used for teas, but it is possible to add some ginger to a variety of beverages and cocktails. Ginger powder can be used as a spice for burgers or salad.

Ginger Teas
Try these different formulations or experiment on your own.

1. Sweetened ginger tea: 1 tablespoon of the grated ginger root, 3 cups of boiled water, honey, brown sugar, or maple syrup according to taste, lemon or apple juice.

2. Pure ginger: Cut a few slices of fresh ginger root and drop into a cup of just-boiled water. Put a pinch of finely chopped ginger in the boiling water, cover the cup, wait 10-15 minutes and drink.

3. Latte: 1 tablespoon of freshly cut or sliced fresh ginger root, a cup of boiling water, 2 cups of milk (it could be soy milk), add honey or maple syrup according to taste.

4. Ginger ale: 2 tablespoons of grated ginger, 1 liter of water, juice from 1 juicy lemon, some ice cubes, brown sugar or honey.

Horseradishes

About Horseradish (Armoracia rusticana, syn. Cochlearia armoracia). Horseradish is a perennial plant of the Brassicaceae family. The plant has a long and narrowing root which is used as a spice. This root has a strong and sharp taste. Horseradishes originated in Asia before later arriving in Europe and spreading to America during colonization. The best place to grow them is where the climate is cool with plenty of sunshine.

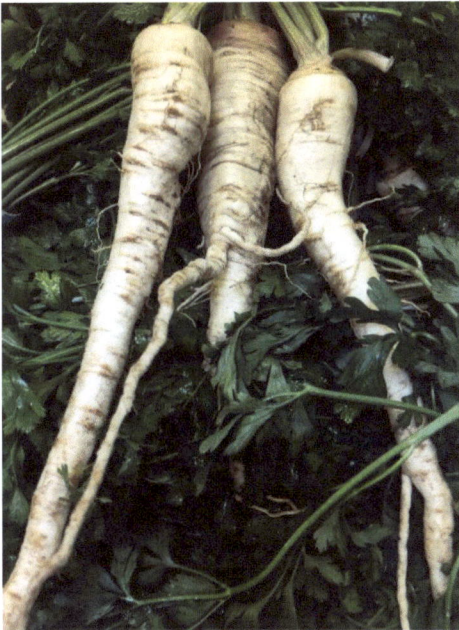

Horseradishes contain minerals, folic acid, vitamin B6, riboflavin, niacin, omega-3, and omega-6. They are rich in vitamin C, which is a potent antioxidant. Horseradishes protect against viral infections. As strong gastric stimulants, they stimulate appetite, improve digestion, stimulate the saliva, stomach, and intestinal glands, and facilitate digestion.

Horseradishes strengthen immunity, stimulate the production of white blood cells, and dilate blood vessels. They are suitable for people with low blood pressure, cure coughs, gastritis, and stimulate urine.

Grated horseradish is used as a spice for flavoring meat, fish, and salad dishes.

Horseradishes do not need to be consumed in large quantities

Industrially prepared horseradishes are available in stores throughout the year. If you grate the root of the horseradish yourself, add vinegar to it after grating to help stabilize the sharpness. Grated horseradish should not be left to stand for a long time as it loses its taste properties.

Spicy Pepper

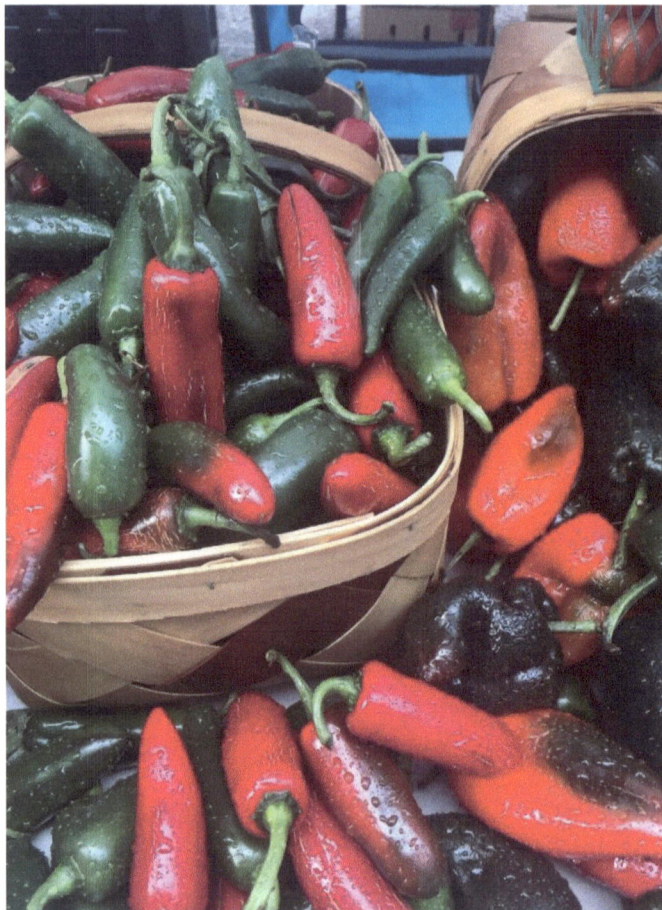

About Peppers: There are about 200 types of peppers in the world, often ranked by their concentration of capsaicin, which is a strong antioxidant. Peppers are unique spices with a rich variety of flavors. In particular, the cayenne peppers (Capsicum frutescens) may be used for food, health, and beauty aid.

Health Benefits of Spicy Peppers: Spicy peppers are rich in vitamins C and E and antioxidants that improve the condition of the epidermis and the skin. They contain anti-inflammatory, anti-allergic, anti-fungal, and anti-irritant properties. They contain vitamins A, B6, C, beta-carotene, magnesium, and potassium.

MEDICAL USES OF SPICY PEPPERS

1. Beautiful facial skin.
If you eat spicy pepper twice a day in your food, your skin will be much more beautiful.

2. Capsaicin inhibits the growth of fatty acids and removes waste from the body. It also activates brain activity.

3. It accelerates metabolism, promotes digestion and gastric juice excretion, and it helps to get rid of excess weight.

4. When capsaicin comes to our body, it combats against microbes, strengthens immunity, stimulates the activity of the cardiovascular system, reduces cholesterol levels, and reduces the risk of thrombus formation.

5. Mood Improvement

When you regularly use chili peppers, you will feel how your mood improves. It is also easier to cope with stressful situations.

6. Peppers heal the throat.

Rinse the throat with water mixed with cayenne pepper powder. Irritation will stop quickly.

7. Lip plumpness

Add a pinch of ground cayenne pepper to a lip balm. Cayenne pepper plumps the lips and brightens their natural color.

8. Hair Strength and Gloss

Mix 25g ground pepper with ½ liter of olive oil. Pour the mixture into a dark, glass bottle and store in a dark place. After 12-15 days you can start using it. Grease the scalp and hair with this mixture, wrap it with a cloth, wait an hour, then wash your head with a shampoo. After constant use of this mixture, the hair will be thick and shiny. Use this formula between weekly or monthly, depending on your results.

It should be borne in mind that the infusion of sharp peppers stimulates hair growth but also irritates the skin. Be careful not to get the infusion into your eyes. Wash your hands after washing your head. If you are going to grease the scalp with the infusion, dilute it with a little water. If the skin does not irritate, the infusion does not need to be diluted.

9. Effects on the blood and circulation

Sharp peppers extend the blood vessels. Capsaicin liquefies the blood and prevents the formation of clots. It is also a natural measure for lowering blood pressure.

10. Aphrodisiac.

Capsaicin has toning qualities; therefore, the Indians took a piece of black chocolate with Cayenne pepper and served it as a husband's dinner before meeting with his woman.

COOKING WITH SPICY PEPPER

Spicy peppers can be added to any dish and provide savory and brightness. For example, add spicy pepper to avocados for a tasty and spicy treat.

A Recipe for a Romantic Evening

Hot Chocolate for Two Persons

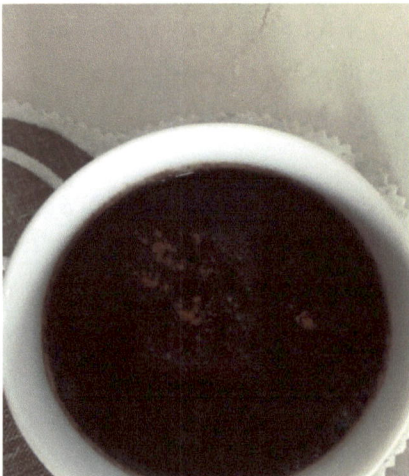

Break 200 g of black chocolate (70% cocoa), into small pieces. Add to 300 ml of heated but not boiled milk. Mix until the chocolate is completely dissolved. Add pinches of cayenne pepper (A very small amount of cayenne pepper powder is recommended). Add cinnamon, ginger, and/or vanilla. This is a wonderful toning drink.

Turmeric

Turmeric (Curcuma longa). Turmeric is a perennial plant of the Zingiberaceae ginger family and is a species of the Curcuma ginger family. This spice is widely used in Indian, Middle Eastern, South American, and Asian cuisines.

It can grow up to 90 cm in height, with large simple leaves. The flower blossoms with green on the bottom and white on the top. There are small tubes in their yellow blossoms. Turmeric supplements come from the plant's rhizomes, which feature rough, brown skin and a dark orange flesh, and available as liquid extract, capsule, and powder forms.

Commonly used in Asian food, you probably know turmeric as the main spice in curry, giving it a distinctive flavor and a yellow color. It has a warm, bitter taste and is frequently used in curry powders, mustards, butters, and cheeses. The root of turmeric is also used widely to make medicine.

It is used as a food coloring agent (E 100) and as a yellow pigment in cosmetics. In India, saris and the garments of Buddhist monks are painted with this substance. Turmeric is also used for weddings and in the contribution to deities (puja) ceremonies.

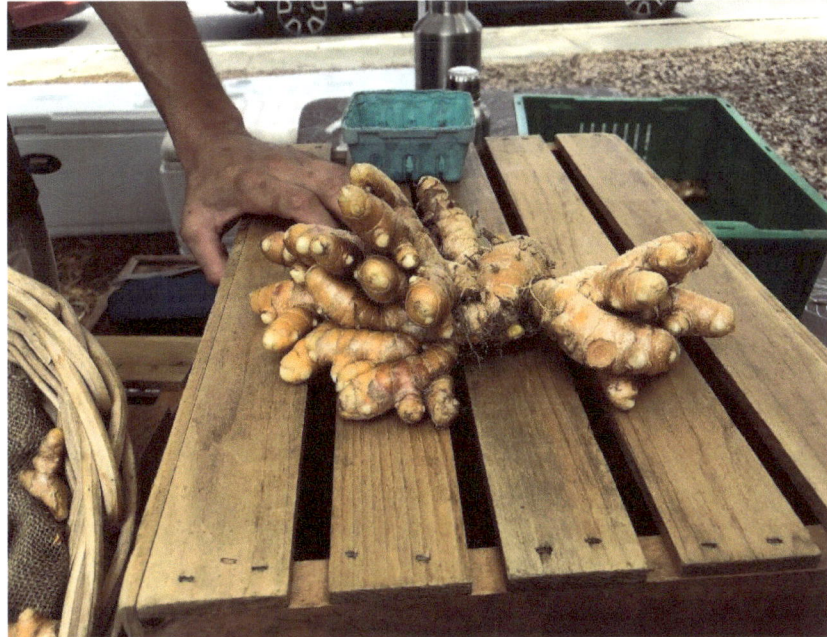

MEDICAL USES FOR TURMERIC

Turmeric is rich in vitamins C, A, B1, B2, B3, and E, as well as micro elements such as iron, calcium, phosphorus, and iodine. Turmeric has antiviral, antifungal, anti-inflammatory, and anti-carcinogenic properties. Due to its antioxidant properties, it helps to remove free radicals from the body.

The main use for Turmeric is to reduce inflammation such as suppressing arthritis pain, joint inflammations, muscle pain, and to relieve chronic inflammatory pain. Due to its antioxidant properties, turmeric is suitable for the treatment of liver diseases.

Other traditional uses include
Regulating gastrointestinal activity and improving digestion
Dissolving fatty meals
Antibiotic properties
Prediabetic and diabetic supplements
Treatment of skin ulcers and prostate cancer
Reduction of cholesterol levels.
Treating cold symptoms
Strengthening the immune system,
Encouraging wound healing
Weight control
Alzheimer's disease protection
Antiseptic ointment
Skin Care – In Indian medicine turmeric is used for the treatment of itching, dermatitis, and allergic rash. They create a paste containing the turmeric and apply it directly to the diseased skin, such as ulcers, eczema, and infected sites.

Dosage:500 mg of curcumin per day

Do not use turmeric to treat bile duct obstruction or if you have bile duct stones. Turmeric should not be used in the treatment of infertility or for the treatment of blood disorders. Large turmeric levels inhibit blood clotting and should not be used if you have gastric ulcers, increased acidity in stomach, pancreatitis, if you are a pregnant or infant-feeding mother, or if you have immune system disorders or allergic symptoms.

RECIPES

Cooking with turmeric: Enrich the diet with this effective spice. Pick up a pinch of turmeric when preparing meat, fish, vegetables, dishes, soups, and stews. To balance out its tartness, add a little low-fat yogurt to the stew. Turmeric is better absorbed when taken with black pepper.

1. **Antimicrobial grease:** Mix one part turmeric with two parts ghee butter. Ayurvedic medicine uses this ointment as an antimicrobial and anti-aging medicine. It also enhances skin tone.

2. **Turmeric and honey tea**
   (Commonly called "Golden Tea" **This tea is not recommended for daily consumption.**)

Ingredients: 1 teaspoon of honey, a pinch of turmeric powder, a few cayenne peppers, water.

Preparation: pour hot, boiled water into a big glass or a cup. Add honey, turmeric powder, and a pinch of cayenne peppers or black pepper.

3. **Omelet with Turmeric**

Ingredients: 2 eggs, 1 tablespoon of milk, a pinch of turmeric powder and black pepper (add a little more turmeric than pepper).

Preparation: Mix eggs, milk, turmeric, pepper, and pour the mass into a heated pan.
This omelet gets a savory taste and a beautiful color.

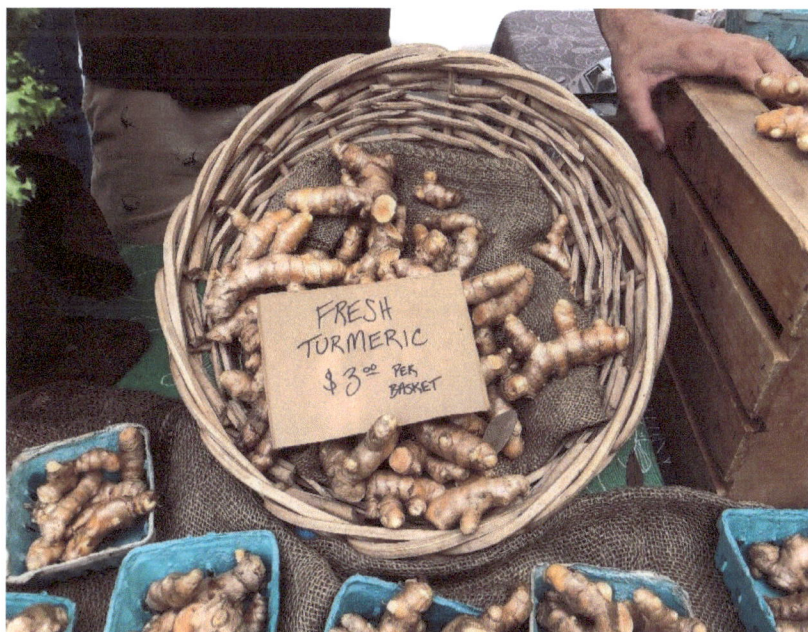

4. Kugel (Potato dish)

Ingredients:
- 15 potatoes,
- 2 eggs,
- 1 onion,
- 5 tablespoons of sunflower oil (it can be replaced with butter - 8 tablespoons or ½ cup),
- 1 tablespoon of natural soy protein (Bragg Liquid Aminos all-purpose seasoning from soy protein),
- 1.5 tablespoons of turmeric powder,
- 1 teaspoon black pepper.
- Salt is not added. Liquid Aminos gives a salty taste.

Preparation: wash the potatoes, peel them, and grate them (with a potato grating machine). Also grate the onion. Put the eggs in the grated mass and add the oil or warmed butter, Liquid Aminos, turmeric powder, and black pepper. Bake in the middle of a preheated oven at 180°C (350 F) for 1.5 hours until the top is beautifully brown.

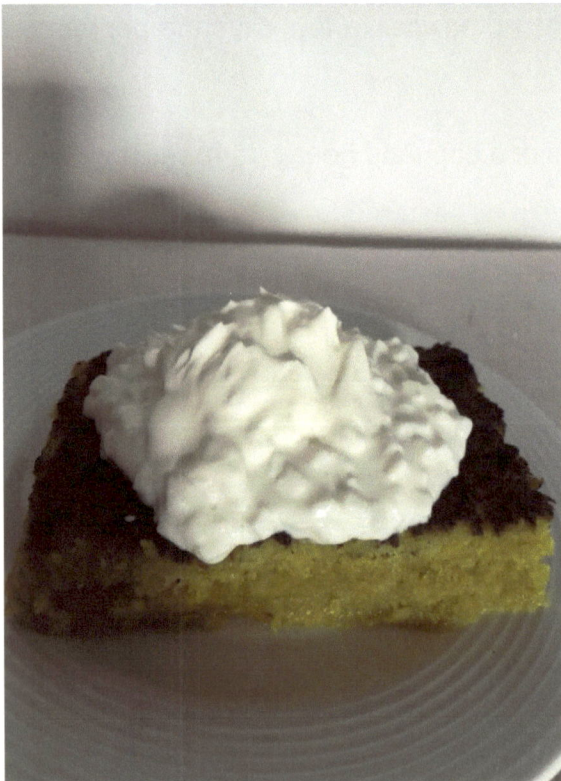

You can serve Kugel with sour cream or curd, apple jam, honey, or maple syrup. You can also mix several ingredients together to make a spicy and colorful kugel topping.

The next day, if you have leftovers, cut into small cubes and fry in a pan with sunflower oil. They will look like glamorous cookies.

CHAPTER 3

ALOE VERA, DANDELION, AND CANNABIS

Nature's crown is made of love. She separates all existences, and all tend to intermingle. She has isolated all things in order that all may approach one another. She holds a couple of drafts from the cup of love to be fair payment for the pains of a lifetime.
– Johann Wolfgang von Goethe, German poet and novelist, 1749-1832.

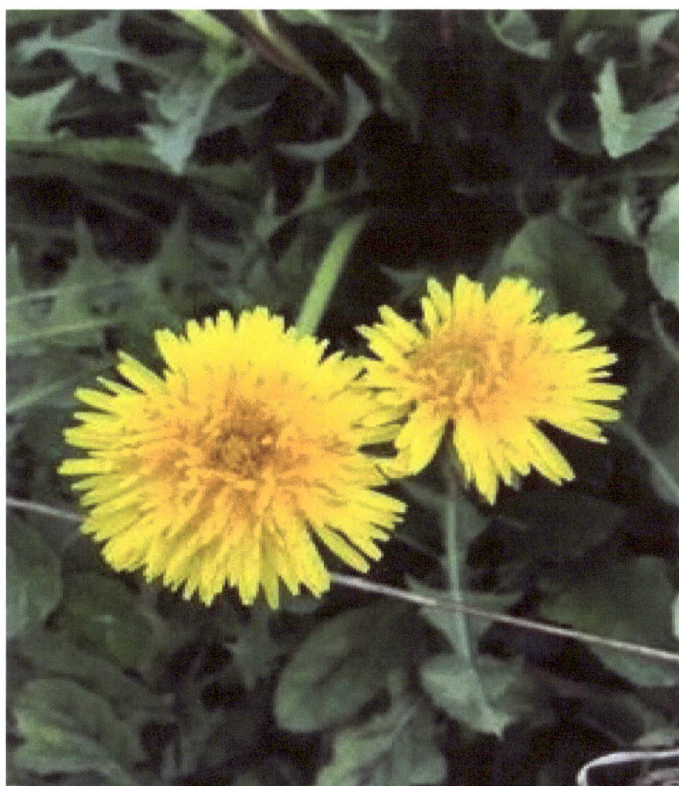

Dandelion

And the dandelion does not stop growing because it is told it is a weed. The dandelion does not care what others see. It says, "One day, they will be making wishes upon me." B. Atkinson, Professor from England. 1944-2017 "The Peaceful Achiever"

Elixir from Juice

Once upon a time, the King of Bavaria (Germany) forced his family to come to the living room in the afternoon where an old manor pharmacist awaited his Majesty with a bottle of fresh dandelion juice. The King insisted every family member drink a small glass of the magic juice. They all enjoyed wonderful health the rest of the summer. This has now become a European tradition.

Dandelion (Taraxacum officinale). The benefits of the dandelion have been known for a very long time, and even Avicenna recommended this plant as a cure for many diseases. Modern specialists agree with the ancient doctor that the dandelion has a unique composition. Carotene present in the dandelion leaves can help improve vision and the health of the skin and mucous membranes.

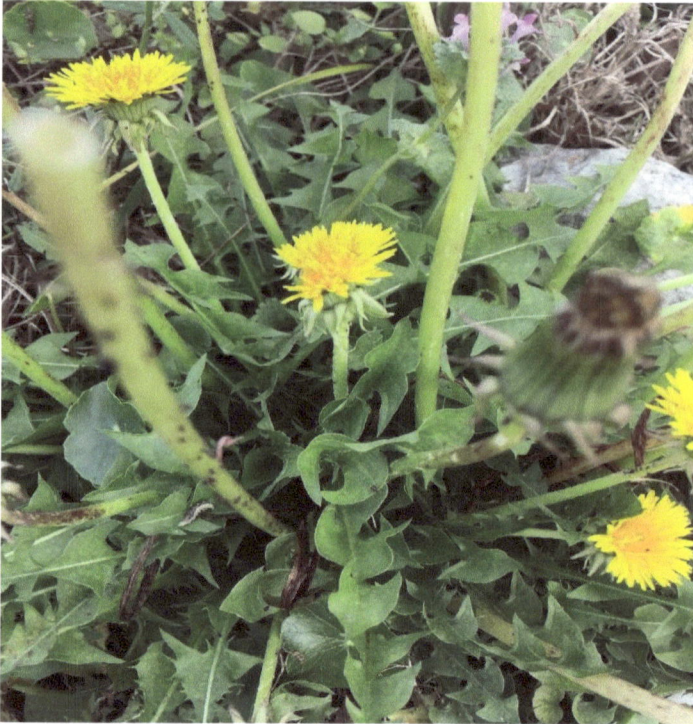

Vitamin C protects the body against infections and aging, vitamin E helps to absorb ascorbic acid and regulates nervous system activity. The roots, leaves, and blossoms all have healing properties. This plant contains useful microelements such as iron, which improves blood composition, and manganese, which is necessary for blood cells, and copper for calming nerves. However, the most important ingredient in the dandelion is the dietary fiber inulin. Inulin reduces the amount of harmful cholesterol in the blood, regulates intestinal microflora, and removes harmful toxins from the body. Inulin is very useful for people with diabetes because this substance is a recognized measure of sugar levels in the body. Also, the most exciting thing is that nobody has genetically modified the dandelion yet.

The dandelion is not a demanding plant, yet it does contain many of the useful elements of the Mendeleev table. They are as follows: potassium, sodium, manganese, aluminum, iron, copper, calcium, and vitamins A, B, E, and C. From ancient times, dandelions have typically been called "life elixirs" which help to relieve pain, stomach acidity, stimulate urine, and perspiration. These elixirs also have an anti-inflammatory and tonic effect. Dandelion leaves provide teeth strength and inhibit the onset of periodontitis.

World professionals esteem dandelion
In France, Austria, the Netherlands, Germany, India, Japan, and the USA, dandelions are grown on special plantations. French people eat them as healing salads, make sauces, use them in marinating, boil them into jam, and make them into wine. Young dandelion leaves practically do not have any bitterness. Exotic jams are made from fresh buds, and excellent beverages can be made from the roots, in a somewhat similar way to coffee.

It is not a Doctor, it is Gold
Dandelions are rich in antioxidants, which protect the body from the harmful effects of free radicals. It has a beneficial effect on the metabolism of salts and fluids in the body.

Folk medical extracts, scrubs, and infusions are made from dandelion roots. They treat the pancreas, thyroid diseases, and increased acidity of the stomach, inflammation of the lymph nodes, and various rashes.

The roots contain natural starch and sugar substitutes and can be used as a diet product for liver and gallbladder diseases. Dandelion cleanses the body from toxins and stimulates bile secretion. It also stimulates the vascular system activities. Avicenna treated patients with liver and heart disease with dandelion juice. He recommended them for blood vessel prophylaxis. In ancient times, herbalists even used it for tuberculosis.

Dandelion blossoms are used for the prevention of fatty liver, cirrhosis, gallbladder stones and to cleanse ducts. They improve liver function, help with gastritis, and improve digestion and appetite. Drinking a concoction of blossoms is recommended for those with high blood pressure and insomnia, and the high level of iron in the blossoms increases hemoglobin levels in the blood. They also help to heal joint infections. It is also good for removing stress, even long-lasting stress, and also for diabetes and thyroid problems.

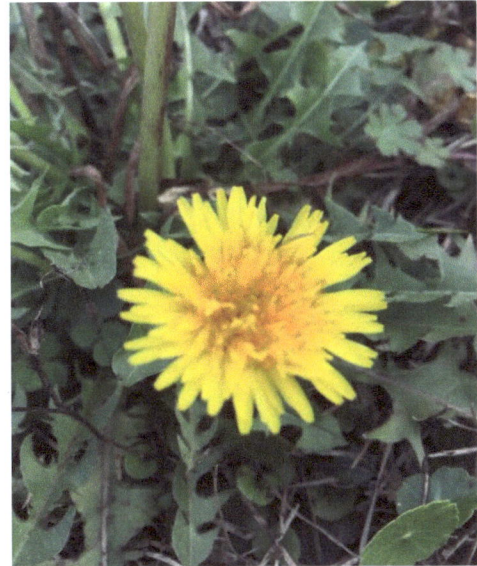

Preparation:
In the early spring, cover an area in the yard thick with dandelions with a black plastic film. After 10 days, the dandelions will grow white instead of yellow and will be less bitter. The roots can be sewn all year round. The best time to pick up flowering dandelions is after a morning rain. Pick the blossoms and leave the stems and pedicles.

Do not use dandelions if you have flu, gall bladder, gut and bile infections, if you are pregnant or a breastfeeding mother, or if you are allergic to them or taking antibiotics.

Ethereal Beauty
The dandelion's ability to eliminate dead cells, moisturize them, and make skin elastic has been used successfully in cosmetology. Nourishing, moisturizing, bleaching, and rejuvenating cosmetics are often made from dandelions. Dandelion juice has been used to bleach the coloration of freckles and pigmented spots. The daily use of cosmetics made from dandelions makes the skin bright and reduce acne. It will help in healing rashes, abscesses, and pimples. Dandelion root powder also heals wounds, ulcers, or burns. It is present in many face masks. Dandelion juice can be applied directly to warts or pigmented spots and rinsed after half an hour (do not use this solution on the face).

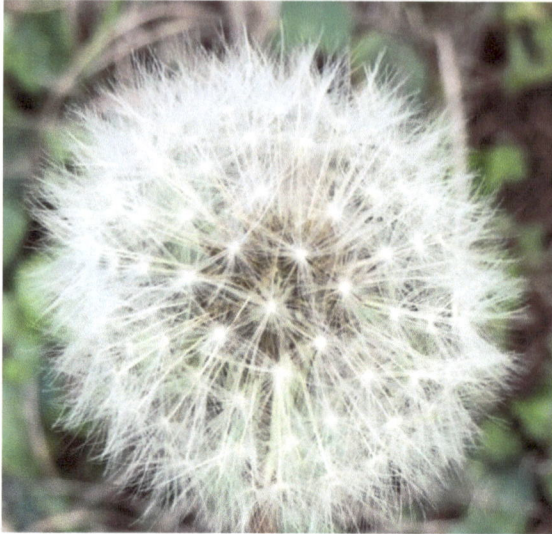

Digestive Tea

Collect dandelions blossoms while they are blooming, avoiding areas near roads, cars, and gas. Cut the blossoms into parts and store in the freezer to use in autumn or winter when there are no yellow sunflower blossoms in the field. Use them to make a tea to stimulate digestion and improve the functioning of the bile and liver.

Dandelion Coffee

Harvest dandelion roots early in the spring, as soon as the first leaflets shoot, or in autumn when the leaves fall (the roots in the fall are more valuable). Scrub the roots with a sponge, trim and dry them. In cold climates, the roots can be dried in a low heat oven at 40°C. Once dried, the roots can be ground in a coffee-mill and made into coffee.

Dandelion Lotion:

An excellent tool for cleansing your face and neck deeply and firmly.

Excavate 3-4 plants together with the roots, stems, leaves, and blossoms. Rinse them well, dry with a napkin, cut them, and place into a clean glass bowl. Next, add vodka (one glass of vodka for one glass of chopped greens), close tightly, and store in a dark place for 10 days. After that, filter the decoction and dilute it with boiled water (half a glass of decoction - one glass of water). Clean face and neck skin with this homemade dandelion lotion twice a day. If the skin is particularly oily, soak a facecloth with the solution and hold it onto the face and neck twice a week for up to five minutes.

Hair strengthening:

Add one tablespoon of dandelion leaves to a glass of boiled water and leave for half an hour to settle. After shampooing, use this as a rinse, letting it soak in for two minutes before rinsing. It will strengthen hair roots and reduce hair loss.

Indigestion:

Add 5 cups of dandelion heads to 1000 ml of water and leave for 8-10 hours to settle. Filter out the solids and add 6 cups of sugar to the liquid. Finally, boil slowly for 1½-2 hours, stirring regularly. Use ½ to one cup for indigestion.

Constipation: Take 2-3 tablespoons of dried crushed dandelion leaves, add 500ml of boiling water. Shake and filter. Store in the refrigerator and drink ½ glass 3-4 times a day half an hour before eating.

Arthritis. The stems are used for the treatment of rheumatism. Finely chop the dandelion stems and mix in powdered sugar. Add 1 teaspoon of the resulting mass to food twice a day.

Liver and Gallbladder Diseases. The washed roots can be cut like carrots. The bitterness of the roots strongly affects the liver, improves the tone of bile ducts and bile secretion, and prevents stone disease. Add 2 tablespoons of crushed roots, to 2 glasses of cold water and soak for about 3 hours. Heat for about 15 minutes at a low temperature. Filter, and drink 1 tablespoon of this decoction 6 times a day about 20 minutes before meals and again 20 minutes after eating.

Bronchitis

Take one part fresh washed dandelion roots, one part honey, and one garlic clove. Grind the roots and mix with honey, then add the garlic. Keep it in a sealed glass container for 2-3 days. During this time the honey will dissolve. It is recommended to consume one teaspoon of this syrup three times a day. This concoction may also help with clearing away blood vessel plaques.

Cough medicine

Rinse thoroughly a handful of dandelion and couch grass roots but don't scrub them. Chop the roots and cook with carrots in a potato soup.

Pesticide

The dandelion has long since been the enemy of a gardener. However, this weed will become a useful helper if you make it a pest control tool. Take a bucket of dandelion leaves, chop finely, and add water. Sprinkle the garden trees with this decoction once a week. Destructive beetles and worms will stay away!

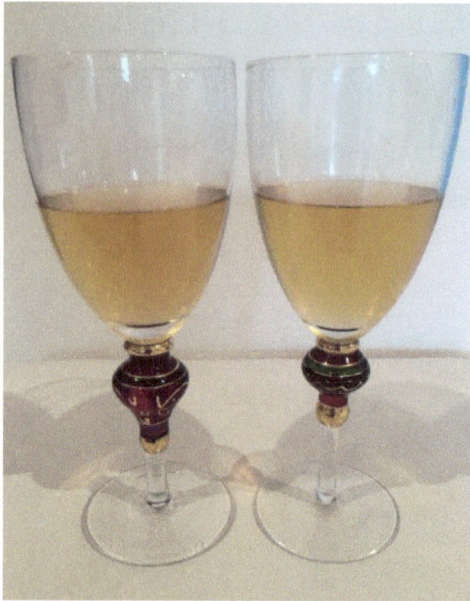

Dandelion Wine

In ancient times, aristocratic women used dandelion wine in order to lose weight—they drank the wine one hour before meals, during dinner, and in the evening, but not more than two ounces (one portion is about 87-90g, per day 280g). They used to wash with dandelion wine so that their skin would not wrinkle but remain firm and youthful. Its effect was much more long lasting than the creams promoted nowadays.

By the way, unusual wine glasses were used for drinking the dandelion wine but without the feet, as the aroma and taste characteristics of the dandelion wine were best revealed by holding the glass placed on the arm and warming it with the heat of one's own hand. When tasting high-quality, freshly-prepared wine at room temperature, you must feel the dandelion's hotness. It is also possible to make a delicious soft drink according to one's own taste.

With the remarkable taste of elegance, let us give our relatives this exceptional wine with an extraordinary flavor.

Dandelion Wine:

About 20 liters of dandelion blossoms (2-3 buckets), 5kg (20 cups) of sugar, 200g raisins (1 cup), 1 kg (5-6) of lemons. Place the fresh dandelion blossoms in a large enameled or wooden container and fill with 20 liters (2 buckets) of boiling water to soak the dandelion blossoms. Leave for 1-2 days.

Pour the liquid into a glass bowl used for wine (a container of 20 liters), add sugar, raisins, and chopped lemons and leave to bubble. You can also put honey instead of sugar (You will need the same amount of honey).

After about a month, when the process has stopped bubbling so after the first fermentation, taste the drink and add more sugar if necessary, or add other ingredients. Use your imagination. After all, the taste itself is a thing of fantasy. After a taste, leave the wine to stand still.

In the autumn, pour the wine into bottles, put them in a dark, cool room and forget it again until spring. When the fields are yellow again with dandelions, invite all your heartwarming friends and enjoy life with them by drinking this light and pleasant dandelion wine.

Dandelion Honey

Ingredients: 200 dandelion blossoms, 1 lemon, 1 l (1000 ml) of water, 1 kg of sugar.

Preparation: Rinse the dandelion blossoms thoroughly, pour into water, and boil for 15-20 minutes. Leave the decomposition for one day at room temperature. Then filter, remove the petals, add sugar and finely chopped lemon to the water and cook for about an hour on a low heat. Thickness will depend on cooking time. Dandelion honey will be yellow in color and will have a pleasant smell.

When making salads with dandelion leaves:

To prevent the leaves from tasting bitter, immerse them in cold water for several hours, or soak in salt water for five minutes and rinse. These techniques may cause the loss of a few of the nutrients.

Dandelion Mixed Salad

The German writer Goethe enjoyed these salads in the spring.

Ingredients: A handful of dandelions, nettles, and sour leaves, parsley, spring onions, borage, dills, 2 hard boiled and crushed eggs, and 2 chopped onion heads.

Preparation: Mix everything and add the sauce, which is made by mixing one glass of fermented milk mixed with salt and pepper and half of a crushed lemon with its peel.

The Sun in the Plate – Dandelion and Walnut Salad

It is extremely easy to make a salad from dandelion and walnuts.

Ingredients: A big handful of dandelion leaves and blossoms, 6 walnuts, and 1 tablespoon of olive oil.

Preparation: Rinse the leaves and blossoms. Chop and mix with chopped walnuts and top with your favorite dressing.

Green Salad

Ingredients: dandelion leaves, radish leaves, borage, sour (or hare cabbage), spring onions, sour cream or oil, and spices.

Preparation: Cut a mixture of a handful of the mentioned greens, pour with oil or sour cream, add your favorite spices, and lemon juice. These salads can be decorated with several dandelion blossoms.

Aloe Vera

Aloe (Aloe vera). Aloe originates from East and South Africa. About 200 types of aloe exist in the world, of which the most commonly used is aloe vera (Aloe vera barbadensis). It is a verdant and perennial plant that can survive up to 100 years. The aloe is a succulent, a plant with thick, fleshy, water-absorbing leaves. When the leaf breaks down or is wounded, the skin heals promptly. When exposed to water, the leaf can more than double in size, accumulating water in order to survive long periods of drought.

The famous therapist Avicenna claimed that drinking this natural miracle juice mixed with wine and honey could cure a variety of diseases, from digestive disorders and joint pains to heart diseases and depression. The medicinal herb flourishes in warm climates where its beneficial properties have been praised for more than 4000 years. In ancient Egypt, the aloe was considered a plant of immortality. The beautiful Cleopatra used it to nourish her body and face.

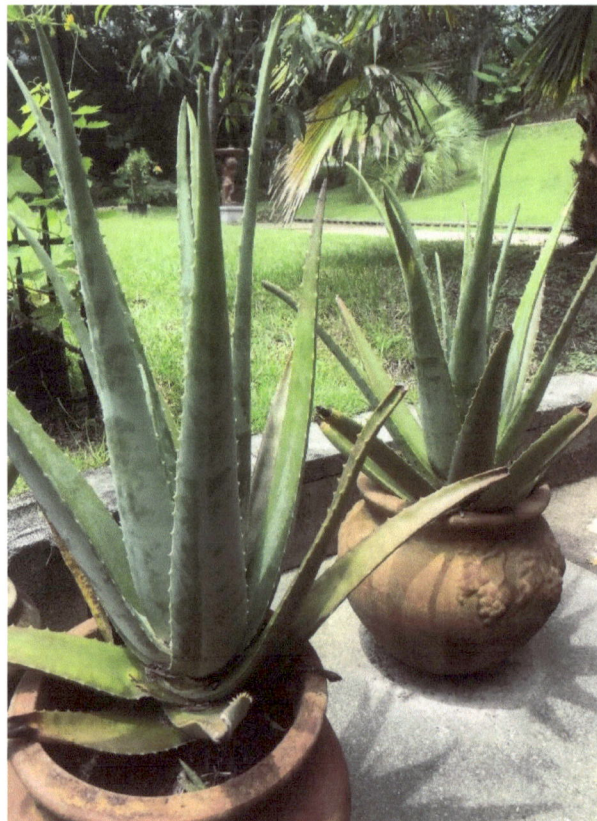

Health Benefits of Aloe

The healing properties of the aloe vera are concentrated in the pulp, not in the cortex which can be peeled off and thrown away. The aloe gel contains over 75 nutrients and vitamins needed for health and vitality, such as polysaccharides, vitamins A, B1, B2, B6, B12, C, E, folic acid, and niacin. Its juices contain plenty of minerals, such as copper, iron, sodium, calcium, zinc, potassium, chromium, magnesium, and manganese. A daily intake of aloe juice enhances the immune system. No side effects have been observed with this medicinal herb which is suitable for both external and internal use.

1. Skin health.

Aloe Vera is available in various lubricants, ointments, and creams and is an excellent moisturizer. Commonly used to treat sunburn, apply the gel directly to the burnt skin with immediate relief. Cut leaves can be used fresh, or stored in a refrigerator. For fungal foot (athlete's foor), apply aloe vera gel to the damaged foot area twice a day. It both heals damaged skin and stimulates the skin regeneration processes. Aloe vera can be used for dry skin care and to treat psyllium and eczema. Its gel illuminates pigmentary stains, destroys scars, maintains the natural beauty of the skin, and reduces itching from insect bites.

2. Aloe Vera treats gastrointestinal diseases.

The internet is awash with information on the properties of aloe vera and its ability to treat heartburn, gastroesophageal reflux ulcers and IBS (Irritable Bowel Syndrome). The miracle cannot be expected immediately as the aloe vera must be used regularly. The most commonly seen improvement is after 2-4 weeks, depending on the severity of the disease. Its enzymes help to digest food and ease minor constipation. Consume 1-2 teaspoons (5 ml-10 ml) of aloe vera juice gel 2-3 times a day for 30 minutes before a meal.

3. Aloe antioxidant properties reduces inflammation, helps with cholesterol, and stabilizes blood sugar

Aloe Vera lotions can be applied onto joints and muscle for arthritis and muscle pain. Aloe reduces the amount of cholesterol and triglycerides and has antidiabetic properties. A number of diabetics managed to significantly lower their blood sugar levels when taking aloe vera for three months. In addition, aloe vera improves blood flow to the limbs in diabetics.

Youth and Good Health Elixir

In a large glass of water, place the juice of ½ lemon or lime, 2-3 large tablespoons of Aloe Vera, 1 tablespoon of honey, and a pinch of Cayenne pepper. Mix and drink in the morning before meals.

For stomach acid issues, drink the above mixture 15-30 minutes before breakfast.
This drink has a magical effect, and each component has the healing properties that are needed for the human body. The drink also helps to quickly eliminate stagnant toxins overnight, in addition to improving lymph circulation, cleansing the blood, strengthening immunity, fighting bacteria and viruses in our bodies, and providing energy.

How to Use the Leaf of Aloe Vera

After washing the leaf, it should be cut along its length and the skin peeled off. Drop the peeled leaf into a blender. Left over juice can be stored in the refrigerator for five days.

Aloe Vera should not be used by pregnant mothers, or those with very sensitive skin. Other contraindications include liver and bile duct diseases, bleeding in the womb, hemorrhoids, and cystitis.

Cannabis

The plant name cannabis (Cannabis sativa) came from the Greek word *kannabis*. Cannabis, also known as marijuana, is one of the world's oldest cultivated plants. Although the earliest written records of the human use of cannabis date from the 6th century B.C., existing evidence suggests that its use in Europe and East Asia started in the early Holocene, about 8,000 B.C. The history of cannabis cultivation in America dates back to the early colonists, who grew hemp for textiles and rope. Hemp fiber was used to make clothing, paper, sails, and rope and its seeds were used as food.

Most ancient cultures didn't grow the plant to get high, but as herbal medicine, likely starting in Asia around 500 BC. However, there's some evidence that ancient cultures knew about the psychoactive properties of the cannabis plant. They may have cultivated some varieties to produce higher levels of THC (Tetrahydrocannabinol) for use in religious ceremonies or healing practice. Burned cannabis seeds have been found in the graves of shamans in China and Siberia dated about 500 BC.

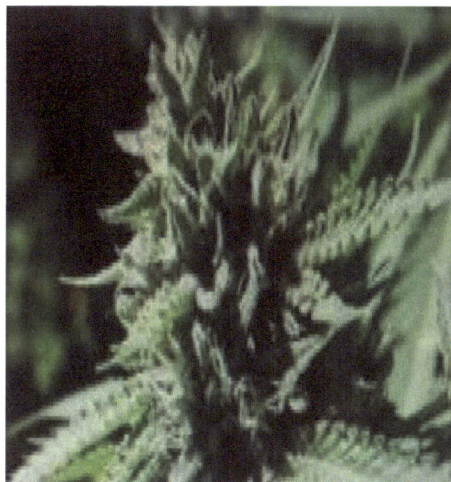

Many 19th-century practitioners ascribed medicinal properties to cannabis after the drug found its way to Europe during a period of colonial expansion into Africa and Asia. For example, William B. O'Shaughnessy, an Irish physician working at the Medical College and Hospital in Calcutta, first introduced cannabis (Indian hemp) to Western medicine as a treatment for tetanus and other convulsive diseases. At approximately the same time, French physician Jean-Jacques Moreau de Tours experimented with the use of cannabis preparations for the treatment of mental disorders. Soon after, in 1851, cannabis was included in the 3rd edition of the Pharmacopoeia of the United States (USP). Subsequent revisions of the USP described in detail how to prepare extracts and tinctures of dried cannabis flowers to be used as analgesics, hypnotics, and anticonvulsants.

Growing concerns about cannabis resulted in the outlawing of cannabis in several states in the early 1900s and federal prohibition of the drug in 1937 with the passage of the Marijuana Tax Act. In response to these concerns, in 1942 the American Medical Association removed cannabis from the 12th edition of U.S. Pharmacopeia. Political and racial factors in 20th century led to the criminalization of marijuana in the United States, although its legal status is changing in many places.

Medical Marijuana facts about Uses, Benefits and Legalities

As of this writing (mid-2018), thirty-one states have legalized the use of medical marijuana. In polls, 70% of the American public supports the legalization of medical marijuana. Several studies show that marijuana has medical efficacy for various conditions, including seizures, post-traumatic stress disorder, bowel diseases, narcotic dependency, and chronic pain. There's also strong evidence medical cannabis can help with muscle spasms, such as those related to multiple sclerosis and muscular dystrophy.

THC may slow the progression of Alzheimer's disease. Research from Israel shows that smoking marijuana significantly reduces pain and tremors and improves sleep in Parkinson's disease. Cannabis may reduce nausea and vomiting from chemotherapy. Less well substantiated studies suggest possible uses in glaucoma, cancer metastasis, sleep disorders, anxiety disorders, narcotic addiction, post traumatic stress disorder (PTSD) and bipolar disorders.

Various authors have expressed different viewpoints concerning psychiatric syndromes and cannabis. While some emphasize the problems caused by cannabis, others promote the therapeutic possibilities. Quite possibly cannabis products may be either beneficial or harmful, depending on the particular case.

Special Precautions and Warnings

1. Pregnancy: As with all medications, cannabis use should be avoided in pregnancy as its effects are unknown.
2. Heart disease: Marijuana might cause rapid heartbeat and lower high blood pressure.
3. Cyclic Vomiting Syndrome: Although cannabis decreases nausea in some people, a few people who use cannabis to excess develop "cyclic vomiting syndrome" which causes non-stop recurrent vomiting, worsened with marijuana use.
4. Lung diseases: There is no evidence that long - term use of marijuana causes any lung effects. However heavy exposure to any smoked substance might have unknown consequences and smokers should consider using filters that cool and clean, such as water pipes. Asthmatics should exercise caution on any inhaled material.
5. Psychiatric: The use of marijuana by those with bipolar or schizophrenic disorders can cause acute exacerbations and should definitely be avoided in these diseases.
6. Possible side effects: Dry mouth, dizziness, increased appetite, memory impairment, lack of motivation and coordination, depression, paranoia, psychological addiction.

Recipe:

Simple Cannabis Cookies.

Cannabutter

Ingredients:
- ½ ounce (14g) marijuana weed,
- 8 ounces (2 sticks unsalted butter),
- four cups water,
- cheesecloth,
- boiling pan.

Preparation: In a medium saucepan bring four cups of water to a boil. When the water is boiling, place the butter in the pan and allow it to melt completely. Once the butter is melted, you can add the marijuana. Try to keep the marijuana floating about 1½ - 2 inches (4-5 cm) from the bottom of the pan. Reduce the heat to simmer for around three hours. You can tell it's done when the top of the mix turns to glossy and thick.

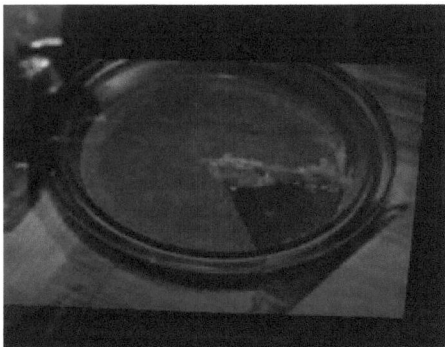

While the cannabis is cooking, set up a heat-proof bowl. Place a double layer of cheesecloth over the top and secure it with elastic, string or tape.

Strain the cannabutter over the bow, carefully trying not to spill. When the saucepan is empty, undo the twine, pick up the cheesecloth from all four sides and squeeze out all of the remaining butter. Allow the cannabutter to cool for about an hour. Place in the refrigerator until the butter has raised to the top layer and is solid. The THC and other properties have attached to the butter.

Run a knife around the edge and lift the butter off. Place upside down in your work surface and scrape off any of the cooking water. The cannabutter is ready to roll.

Cookies with cannabutter

Ingredients:
- 1 cup of flour,
- 1 teaspoon of brown sugar (according to taste),
- ¼ teaspoon of baking soda,
- pinch of salt,
- ½ cup cannabutter (cannabis infused butter) or less,
- ⅓ cup unsweetened chocolate chips (according to taste),

- 2 teaspoon of vanilla extract,
- 1 egg.

Preparation: Preheat the oven to 325 degrees F, (165 degrees C). Grease cookie sheets with butter, or line it with parchment paper.

Sift together the flour, baking soda and salt, then set aside. In another medium bowl, cream together the cannabutter and brown sugar until they are fluffy. Make sure that the cannabutter is at room temperature before mixing in the sugar. Add a well beaten egg and the vanilla extract into the sifted ingredients until just blended. Stir in the chocolate chips. Scoop the dough into the prepared cookie sheet, about one or two tablespoons at a time. Bake for 10 minutes for 1 tablespoon size, up to 17 minutes for larger cookies, judging by the appearance of the cookies being lightly toasted.

Cool on baking sheets for a few minutes.

WARNINGS

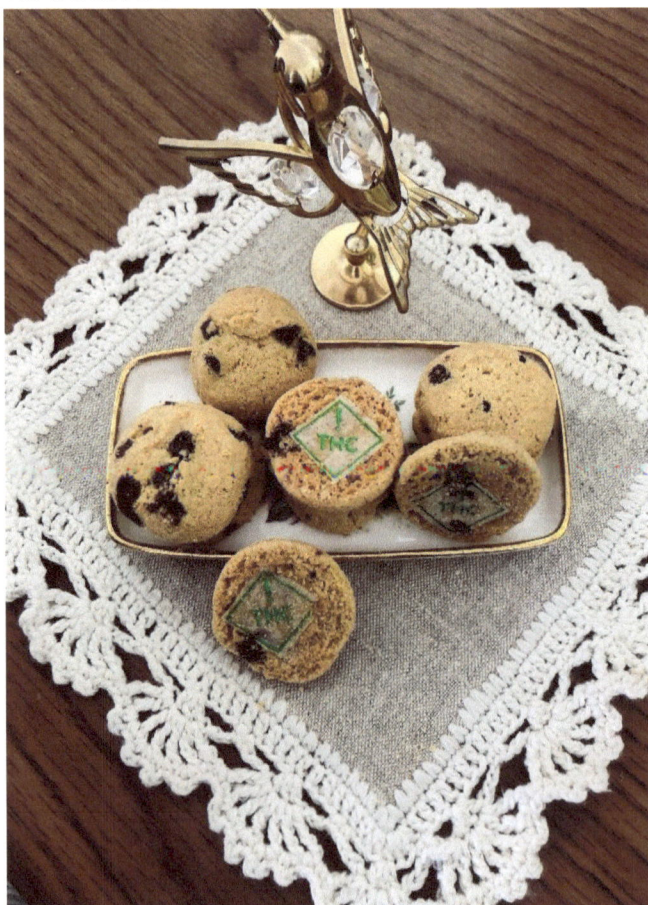

Use caution when eating marijuana cookies. Marijuana infused cookies can produce a more intense, longer lasting high than smoking, so you might want to try eating only ¼ to ½ of a small cookie to start and then wait to see how it affects you.

Cannabis is illegal in some states. Check your local laws.

Be sure to store these and any other marijuana edibles in a safe location with clear labeling to prevent unintended consumption.

CHAPTER 4

HEALING BERRIES

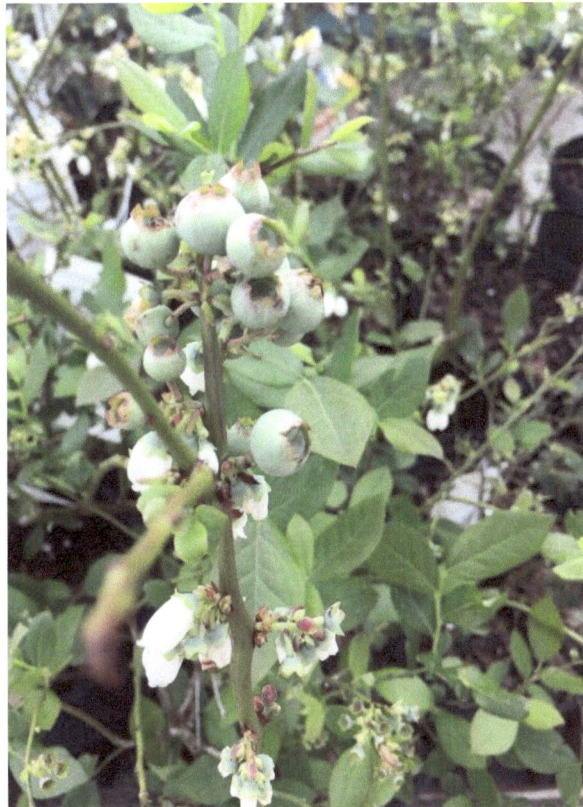

The glory of gardening: hands in the dirt, head in the sun, heart with nature.
To nurture a garden is to feed not just on the body, but also the soul.
-- Alfred Austin, British Poet, 1835-1913.

Happiness is a bowl of fresh berries.

Berries, the most delicious summer vitamins, top the healthy nutrition pyramid. Berries are a great alternative to sweets; not only are they delicious, but they are also useful. Adults should consume 8-12 oz. of fresh berries per day. Five strawberries contain the same amount of vitamin C as can be found in one orange. Eat berries as naturally as possible, without sugar, and in small servings. Make sure to not overload the stomach.

Dig into a variety of berries regularly to reap the "total body" benefits of high nutrient content. To preserve the vitamins in fruits, keep them away from the three natural destroyers: heat, light and oxygen.

Although rare, there are people who are allergic to berries, and of course, those people should not eat them. Otherwise ENJOY!

Cranberries

Cranberries (Vaccinium oxycoccus or in North America, Vaccinium macrocarpon). The healing properties of cranberries have been recognized for centuries. The ancient North American Indians used cranberries for wound healing, as well as loss of appetite, digestion, the treatment of blood disorders, and scurvy.

Cranberries are rich in organic sugars; fructose and glucose; dietary fiber; vitamins C, B1, B2, PP, K, and E; carotene; minerals such as phosphorus, potassium, calcium, phosphorus, iron, manganese; and quite a lot of iodine.

Health Benefits of Cranberries

Urinary Tract Health: Cranberries protect against bladder inflammation and kidney diseases. An ancient belief about cranberries was recently officially confirmed by "Critical Reviews of Food Science and Nutrition." The performed studies found that the acids contained within cranberries kill bacteria such as E-coli, which adhere to the walls of the urinary tract and cause inflammation. They also serve as a preventive measure to avoid the formation of kidney stones.

Digestion: Cranberry-based acids partially destroy the H-pylori bacteria in the stomach that are blamed for gastric ulcers. Rich in antioxidants and fibers that improve digestion, cranberries restore intestinal microflora and stimulate pancreatic secretion. Cranberry juice helps to restore intestinal microflora after the use of antibiotics.

Cardiac: Cranberries reduce the risk of heart attack by lowering the bad cholesterol (LDL) and reducing blood pressure and anemia.

Rheumatism: Warm baths made from cranberry stems and leaves are a great remedy for treating rheumatism, reducing salt accumulations, and eliminating toxins.

Other benefits: Cranberries protect your teeth from breakage and prevent gum disease. Cranberries strengthen memory, particularly in the elderly. The antioxidants can lower the eye pressure in glaucoma and improve certain rashes. I recommend drinking cranberry

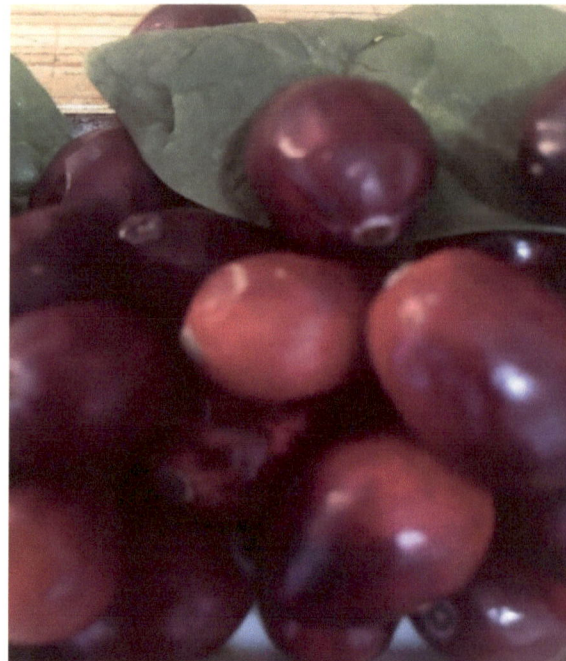

juice during bouts of severe coughing, for chronic inflammation of the kidneys, angina, and heavy headaches. In folk medicine, the cranberry is used to treat scurvy.

When it is better not to use cranberries: Some studies have shown that cranberries can enhance the effect of blood-thinning medicines. Therefore, it is better to avoid cranberries when using these medicines. Consult your family doctor before ingesting cranberries if you are taking similar or related medication.

Popular Recipes for Cranberry Mixes

Cranberry Mixture to Improve Blood Vessels

Ingredients: Take 1kg (4 cups) of cranberries, 200g (4-5 heads) of garlic, ½ liter (500 ml) of fresh unfiltered honey.
Preparation: Grind the cranberries and garlic, mix together, and keep for about 12 hours before adding honey. Make sure everything is mixed very well and eat 1 tablespoon twice a day before meals. This procedure is recommended in autumn and spring.

Mashed Cranberries with Sugar

Ingredients: 1kg (5 cups) of cranberries, 1kg (4 cups) of sugar (preferably brown, although honey can be used as an alternative), 1kg honey. If the jam is too acidic, add more sugar or honey.
Preparation: Cranberries must be clean, fresh, and ripe. Grind the cranberries and add the sugar or honey. Unless you plan to eat them promptly, bring to a boil over moderate heat, stirring occasionally. Reduce heat and simmer, uncovered, for 20 minutes. Put into sterilized (oven-cooled or boiled in hot water) jars. Store the mashed cranberries in a refrigerator. This jam is healthy and delicate, and vitamins are preserved.
Cranberries have low calories—one cup of these berries has 44 calories.
This jam perfectly suits poultry dishes.

Dried cranberries: add to oats porridge, use for various baked things like pies, cookies, cakes. Add to salad, various cocktails.

Blueberries

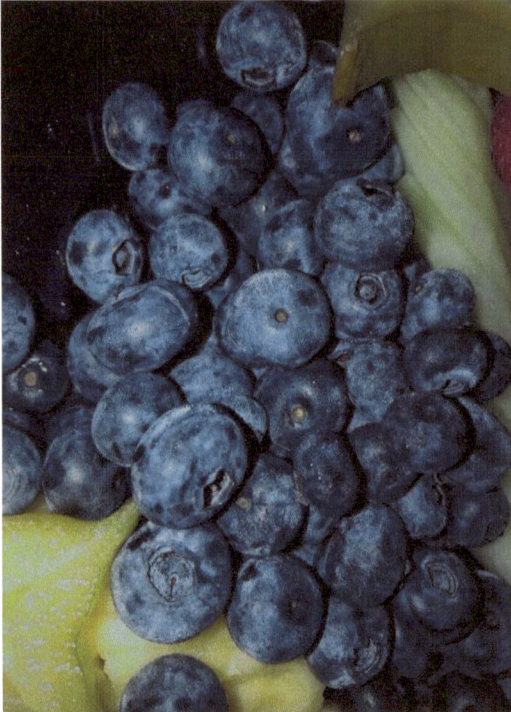

Blueberries (Vaccinium corymbosum or myrtillus). Blueberries are the second most commercially important crop in the United States, and this country is the largest producer of the blueberry.

Blueberries have low calories, 100g blueberries = 54 kcal. They are rich in fiber and have a high pectin content. Moreover, blueberries are excellent antioxidants and a rich source of vitamins C and E, which act as antioxidants, iron, and other minerals and microelements.

If blueberries are fresh frozen, their taste and appearance will be almost unchanged when defrosted.

Health Benefits of Blueberries

Eyes: Blueberries improve vision, stop cataract development, have a positive effect on the blood vessels of the retina and help to prevent retinal bruises. They also reduce eye fatigue.

Diabetes and Inflammation: Blueberries reduce the amount of sugar in the blood, thus making them suitable for diabetics. Blueberry leaves are present in the mixture of herbs against diabetes. They prevent aging, suppress inflammations, and improve and strengthen immunity.

Digestive: Blueberries help the body to recover and heal acute and chronic gastrointestinal diseases. They are suitable for diarrhea, as well as decreased acidity in the stomach. Moreover, they improve digestion and help to regulate intestinal activity.

Other: They are suitable for the treatment of cardiovascular disorders. gout, rheumatism, anemia, kidney, and help with coordination and movement, restore body cells, improve memory, and muscle strength. Blueberries dissolve stones formed in the gall bladder, kidney, or urinary bladder. Blueberries even help to fight against anthrax, which, hopefully will never come up!

Frozen Blueberry Cocktail

This healthy beverage contains extremely high levels of antioxidants and can be taken during lunch-time, used as a snack, for breakfast, or served as a dessert with a biscuit or a warm muffin.

Ingredients: 300g (1.5 teaspoons) of frozen blueberries, 2 tablespoons of lemon juice, 2 tablespoons of honey, 2¼ cup 2% fat milk, a pinch of cardamom.

Preparation: Remove the blueberries from the freezer and leave them to defrost for 30 minutes at room temperature. Mix the defrosted blueberries with an electric blender and add lemon juice, honey, and milk. Add a little cardamom before serving.

It is not recommended to consume too many blueberries as doing so can cause constipation.

Canning Jam, From Preparing the Jars to Testing the Seal.

1. Fit a large pot with a rack, or line with a folded kitchen towel. Fill 2/3 with water and bring to a boil. Add canning jars and boil for 10 minutes. Jars may be left in warm water in the pot until ready to be filled. (Alternatively, you can sterilize jars by running them through a dishwasher cycle and leave them in there until ready to fill).

2. Place canning rings in a small sauce pan, cover with water and bring to boil. Turn off the heat and add lids to soften their rubber gaskets. Rings and lids may be left in the water until jars are filled.

3. Remove warm jars from the pot and bring water back to a boil. Ladle hot jam into jars just up to the base of neck, leaving ½ inch at the top.

4. Wipe jar rims clean with a damp towel. Place lids on jars, screw on rings and lower jars into the pot of boiling water, the water should cover the jar; if not, add more. Boil jars for 10 minutes. Transfer jars to a folded towel and allow to cool for 12 hours; you should hear a pinging sound as they seal.

5. Test the seals by removing and lifting the jars by the flat lid. If the lid releases, the seal has not formed. Unsealed jars should be refrigerated and used within a month, or reprocessed. To reprocess, reheat fillings to the boiling point (as in step 3), then continue as before.

Refrigerated jams will last for weeks, maybe even a few months, when kept cold and tightly sealed. You can also freeze the jams for up to six months before they start to lose their texture.

Strawberries

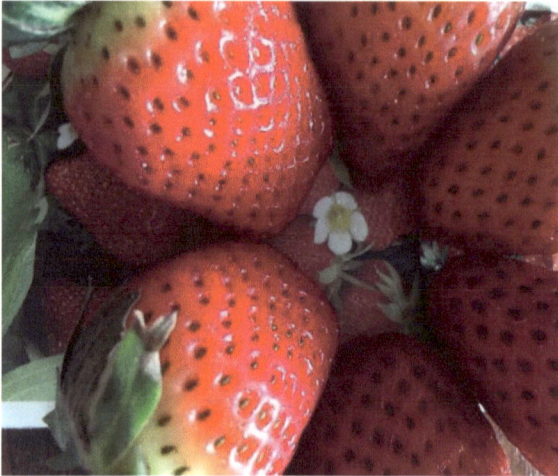

Strawberries (Fragaria x ananassa) are grown on a triticale perennial herbaceous plant that belongs to the strawberry tribe. Strawberries were first bred in the French region of Brittany in the 1750s. Strawberries have a bright red color and the berries are large and juicy. Strawberries can be made into jams, juices, or candies, and makes an excellent wine. They are rich in flavonoids, vitamins, minerals, and strong antioxidants. It is undoubtable that the strawberry has one of the most popular and refreshing tastes on the planet.

Health Benefits of Strawberries

Strawberries have many antioxidants that help protect against heart disease, diabetes, neurological disorders, and the aging process. They also improve brain activity, protect against strokes and intestine constipation, and maintain intestinal cleanliness. Additionally, strawberries help to protect against depression.

The use of strawberries is associated with the prevention of a number of forms of cancer, such as breast, large intestine, skin, and prostate. It is recommended to consume lots of strawberries if you suffer from high blood pressure.

Using strawberries in our diet

There are a number of ways to incorporate strawberries into your diet. For example, you can add a few strawberries to plain yogurt or a chicken salad, or add them to fruit cocktails with other berries. If the cocktail is sour, add a little honey. You can also make strawberry preserves or marmalade. A good idea is to mix frozen strawberries with banana, milk, and ice, to make a delicious and fast fruity cocktail. Another option is to mix strawberries into a spinach salad with feta cheese and walnuts.

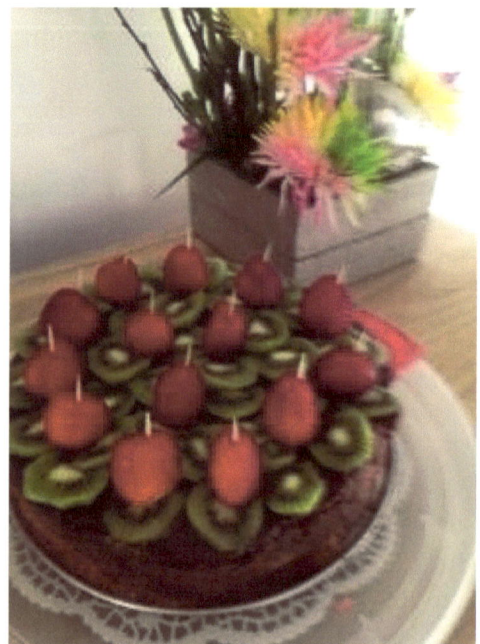

Here are other ideas for Desserts with Strawberries:

A simple bowl of fresh berries in a glass, surrounded by rose petals, makes an excellent "I Love You."

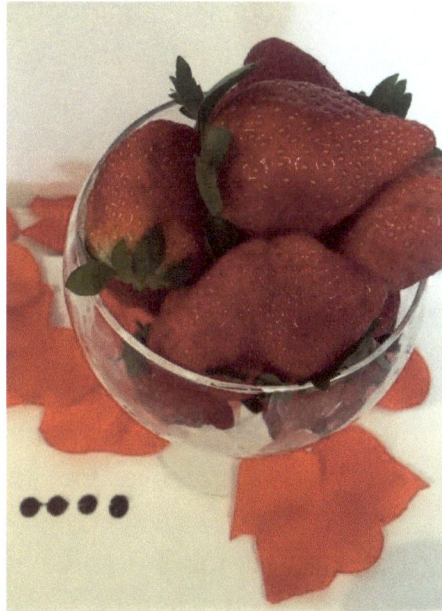

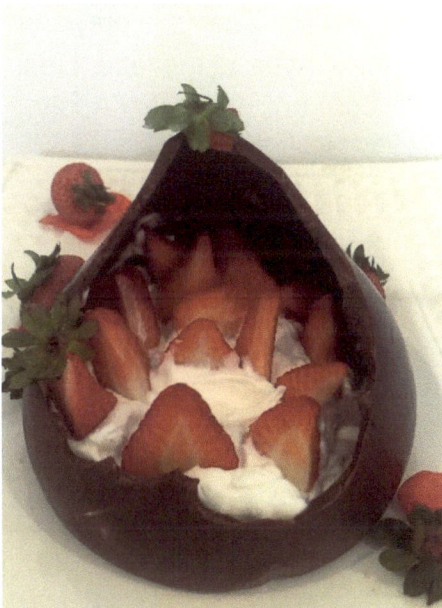

Break open a giant chocolate Kiss, spoon in a layer of yogurt, and decorate with slices of strawberries for a scrumptious and attractive burst of love.

Facial masks from strawberries

A strawberry mask nourishes, strengthens, whitens, and cleanses your facial skin.

Strawberry Face Mask for all types of skin. Chop some strawberries and mix with a tablespoon of sour cream. Spread on your face and leave for 20 minutes.

Strawberry Face Mask for normal skin. Take 2 tablespoons of mashed strawberries and 1 tablespoon of vegetable oil or honey. The mass must be of a liquid consistency. Spread on the face and leave for 15-20 minutes.

Strawberry Face Mask for sensitive skin Crush 2 teaspoons of strawberries and mix with 2 tablespoons of curd or sour cream (without salt). Wear this mask for 15-20 minutes.

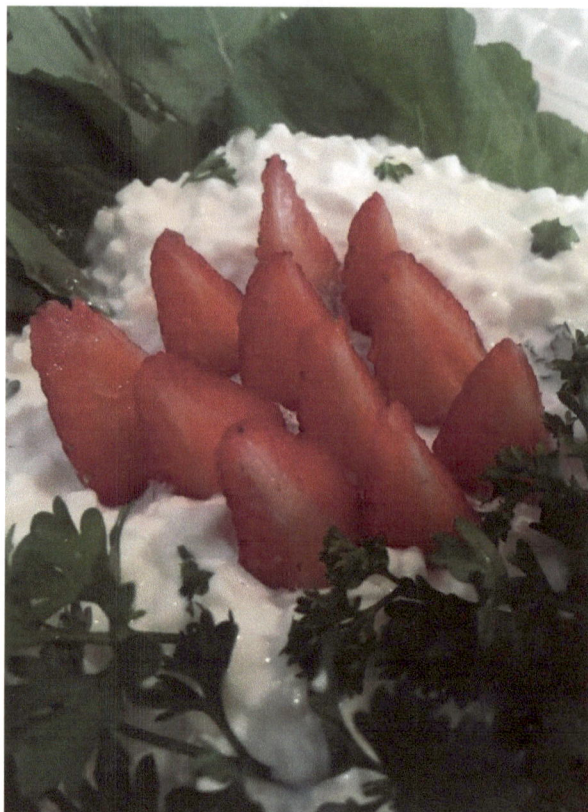

Tips: Your face must be perfectly clean before applying these masks. They are prepared immediately before use. Do not rub around the eyes, apply a thick layer on the face, clean the mask with a cotton swab, and wash the remainder with cool boiling water. Apply a tonic to a clean face and grease the nourishing cream.

Raspberries

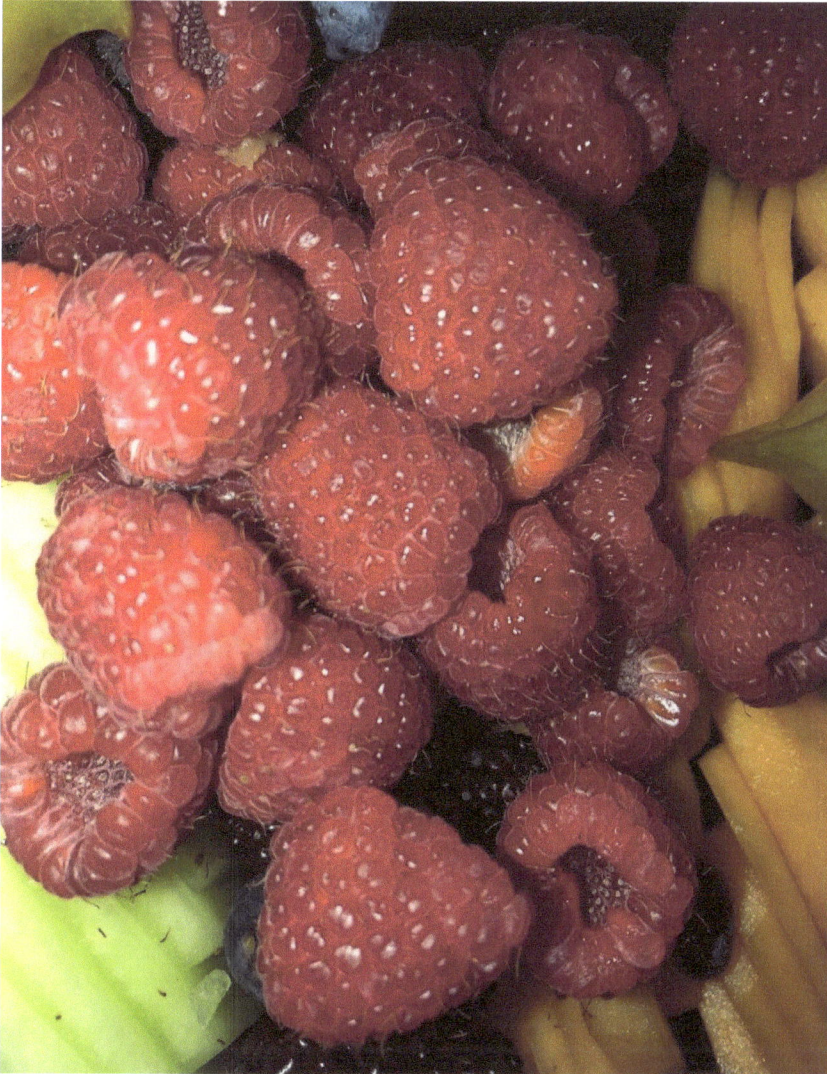

Raspberry (Rubus idaeus). With a very low-calorie index, raspberries have a unique composition of vitamins and antioxidants and are the world's most consumed berries, with Europe being the leading producer. In the United States, raspberries rank as the third most popular berry for fresh use after strawberries and blueberries.

Health Benefits of Raspberries

Raspberries decrease the risk of obesity, heart disease, and the decline in cognitive ability related to aging. Their consumption results in a lower risk of cardiovascular disease, while it also slows down many types of cancer, diabetes, stroke, hypertension, and gastrointestinal disease. Raspberries lower the blood pressure, keep the eyes healthy, inhibit atherosclerosis, and improve digestion, and they are suitable for the treatment of liver diseases.

Blackcurrants

Blackcurrants (Ribes nigrum). Blackcurrants are called "the forbidden fruit" in the United States. Dried blackcurrants are a nutritional powerhouse. They are low in fat, cholesterol free, and high in protein with each cup of dried currant containing 5.88 grams of protein. They are also rich in dietary fiber, copper, manganese, potassium, antioxidants, and vitamins. Poland is the world's leader in the production of currants.

Health Benefits of Blackcurrants.

The blackcurrant is a vitamin superstar. To illustrate, blackcurrants boost the immune system and lower the blood pressure. They also keep joints healthy, reduce arterial plaque, provide assistance to the heart, smooth the skin, and slow the progression of glaucoma. Overall, blackcurrants are wonderful prophylactic tools against cardiovascular problems, Alzheimer's disease, and even malignant tumors. It is known that blackcurrants prevent the development of diabetes and the weakness of intellectual abilities among aging people. They are also useful for the treatment of kidney, liver, and respiratory diseases. These berries should not be forgotten during the progression of atherosclerosis.

Side effects: Blackcurrants and seed oil supplements have been known to cause some side effects, such as soft stool, mild diarrhea, and intestinal clotting. These supplements are not recommended for those who have bleeding disorders or those about to have surgery.

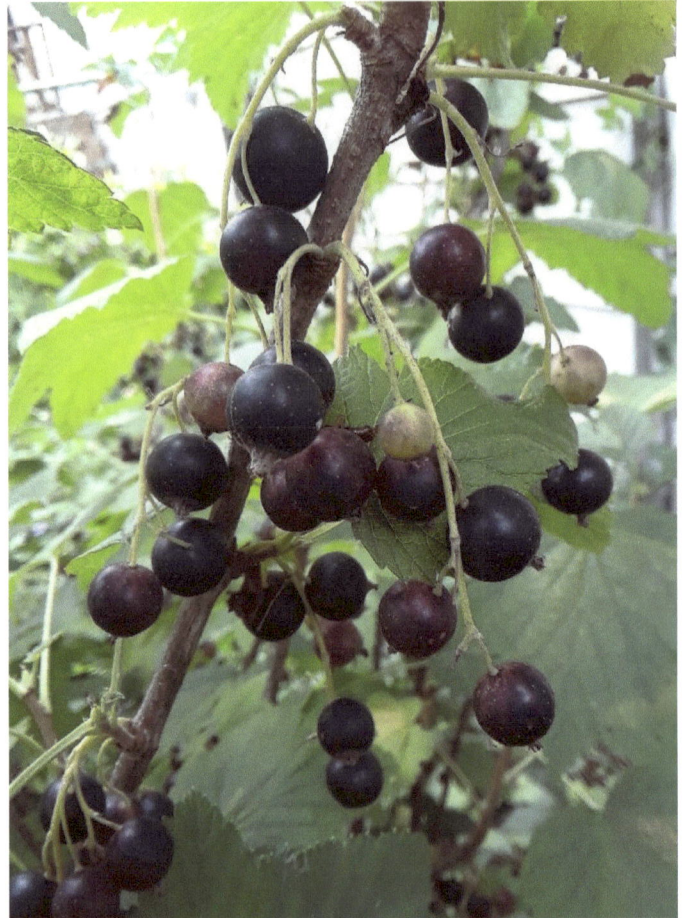

Redcurrants

Redcurrant (Ribes rubrum). Similar to blackcurrants, the redcurrant is a powerhouse of essential vitamins, minerals, and antioxidants that are key to looking youthful, feeling great, and maintaining a healthy and well-nourished body.

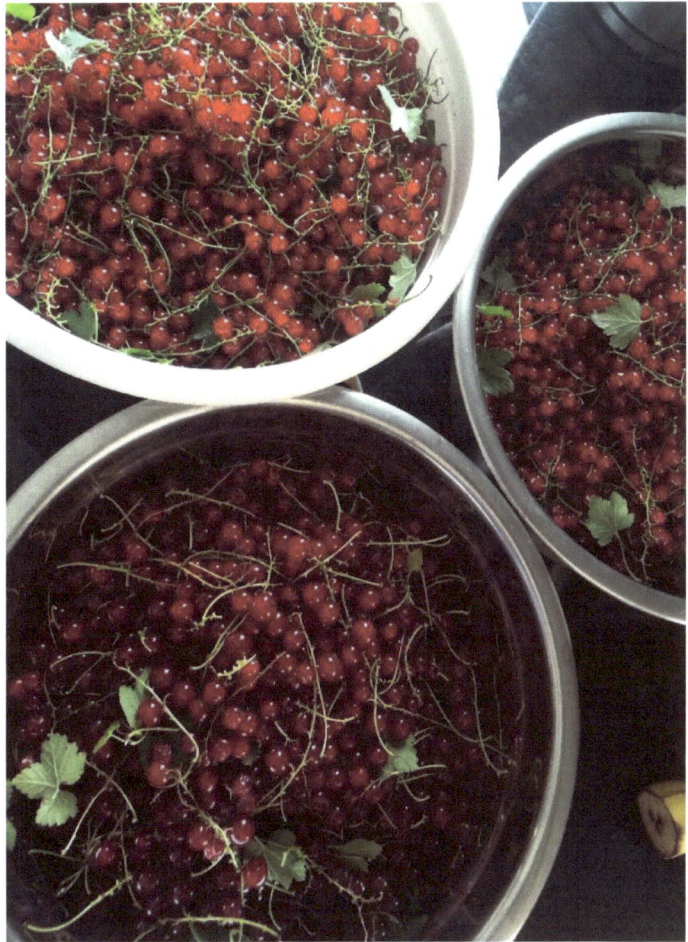

Health Benefits of Redcurrants

They are rich in iron, boost the blood, strengthen the immune system, and prevent free radical damage in body cells. They contain nutrients essential for the formation of red blood cells, promoting regular bowel movement, and reducing acidity in the stomach. The active substances of redcurrants tone the cardiovascular system, regulate the blood pressure, reduce the risk of stroke, maintain adequate blood sugar levels, help with atherosclerosis, rheumatic fever, gout, bronchitis, and gastritis, and they are great for the kidneys. These berries play a key role in normalizing blood clotting and are very important for the prevention of infections.

Redcurrant preparations are used for the treatment of avitaminosis and anemia, and to stop bleeding from the gums or nasal mucosa.

Side effects: Redcurrant juice is a natural laxative, so if drank in excess, this quality can be magnified and could result in diarrhea. Otherwise, red currant juice is suitable for human consumption.

Cherries

Cherries are rich in antioxidants, fiber, vitamins, and carotenoids, each of which may help play a role in the prevention of cancer.

Health Benefits of Cherries

Cherries help to reduce the inflammation of gout, support healthy sleep, arthritis pain relief, reduce belly fat, reduce post-exercise muscle pain, and lower risk of stroke. Cherries activate the body's defensive forces and promote the healing of wounds and the formation of new tissues. They also destroy poisons accumulated in connective tissue, improve the secretion of waste, and improve the functions of digestive organs. In addition, cherries improve the appetite, are suitable for the treatment of anemia, inflammation of the respiratory system, constipation, and reduce thirst and facilitate expectoration.

Side effect: If you eat cherries as part of a very high-fiber diet, you may experience intestinal gas, abdominal cramps, or bloating.

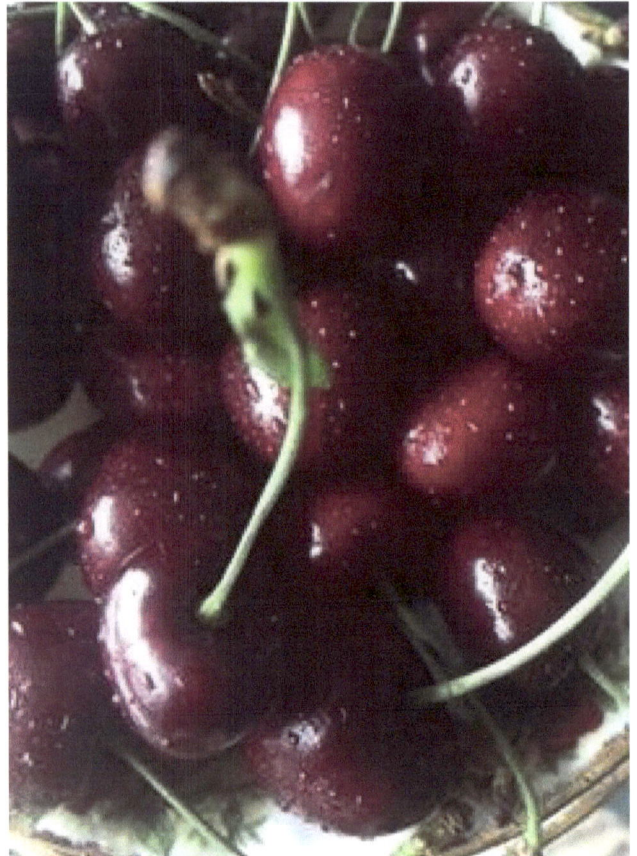

CHAPTER 5: Leafy Vegetables

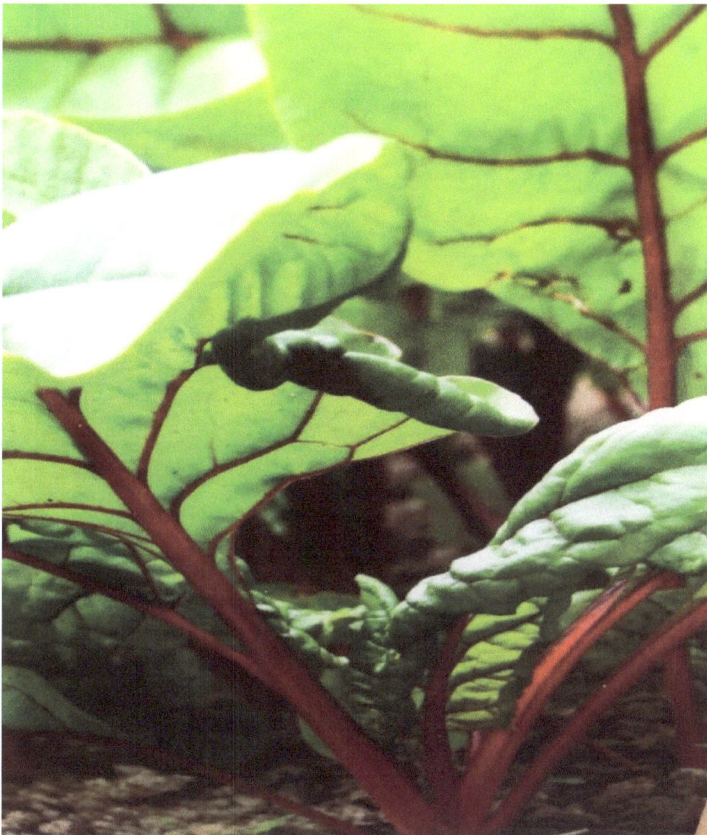

Go vegetable heavy. Reverse the psychology of your plate by making meat the side dish and vegetables the main course. Colors equal healthy. Healthy equals happy.
— *Bobby Flay.*

Every person should incorporate more than 500g of vegetables into their daily diet. Grain crops take first priority, while fruits and vegetables must be a close second. Therefore, cereals, fruits, and vegetables should form the biggest part of the diet. Make meat the side dish and vegetables the main dish. In order to encourage consumption of vegetables, arrange them attractively on the plate when served.

What the colors in your fruits and vegetables provide:

Red color. (Apples, beets, radishes) Red fruits and vegetables are full of antioxidants that protect the skin from the harmful effects of ultraviolet rays, reduce the risk of cardiovascular diseases, and inhibit the development of some oncological diseases. They also prevent memory impairment and reduce the chance of heart attacks.

Orange and yellow colors. (Carrots, corn, oranges) Orange fruits and vegetables greatly improve the immune system. They are rich in carotenoids that are processed into vitamin A in the body and improve the appearance of the skin and help night vision.

Green color. (Celery, spinach, kale) Green vegetables are rich in fiber and low in calories. Eat them with fish and low-fat meats. Chlorophyll, which is rich in green vegetables, is considered the most effective ingredient in the prevention of most cancers. Green plants are essential for dental and bone health. Green fruits and vegetables will help you lose weight without resorting to fasting or other strict diets.

White and pink colors. (Turnip, parsnip, yam) Fruits and vegetables of this color may not look very attractive, but they contain a lot of antioxidant "mines." They reduce the amount of bad cholesterol, lower blood pressure, and reduce the risk of vascular diseases and the development of malignant tumors.

Purple color. (Rutabaga, grapes, eggplant) Purple fruits and vegetables are full of herbal components that reduce the development of malignant tumors, prevent strokes and heart disease, and improve memory. They have a high antioxidant content. However, eggplants and red cabbage have less useful substances than blueberries or healthy berries of the same color, and their dishes are usually cheaper.

Cabbages and Cauliflowers

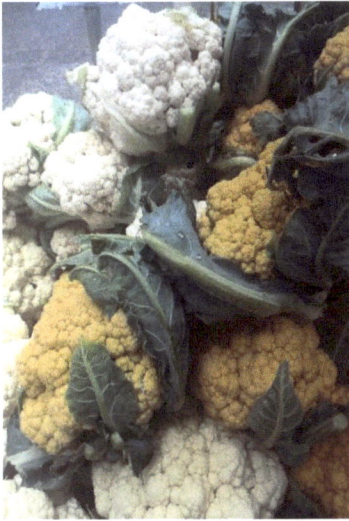

Cauliflowers (Brassica oleracea). The cauliflower belongs to the Brassicaceae family. Cauliflowers spread throughout Western Europe during the 16th-17th centuries, along with cabbages and broccoli. They can be eaten cooked, baked, or consumed raw, and are rich in vitamins and minerals. In addition, the cauliflower is an excellent source of fiber and omega-3 fats, as well as other nutrients. The color of the cauliflower is white, and it has a delicate taste, so it can be prepared or mixed with other foods in various ways. It is recommended to eat cabbages at least twice a week and even better, to eat them four to five times a week.

Health Benefits of Cabbages

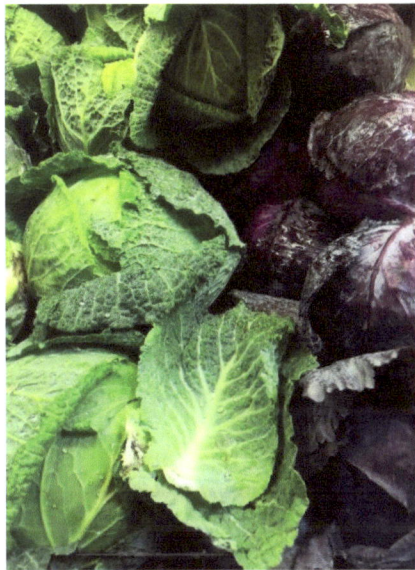

Scientists have noticed that Polish women living in their country rarely suffer from breast cancer, though once Polish women have migrated to the United States, their breast cancer rates rise to the level of other American women. This "Polish Paradox" turns out to have a simple explanation. In America, Polish women have markedly decreased their intake of sauerkraut.

Cabbage is a very strong antioxidant that neutralizes the effects of aggressive radicals. These abundant antioxidants not only prevent breast cancer, but also the formation of malignant tumors in other organs, notably the lungs, the bladder, the large intestine, and the stomach.

Cauliflowers, Brussel sprouts, white cabbages, red cabbages, and broccoli also have the anti-oncological power, with sauerkraut the most effective. It is recommended to eat them as often as possible, so we can improve our health.

Cabbage can also help certain kinds of headaches, but only by consuming it, not by putting a cabbage leaf on your forehead.

Cabbages are not recommended to eat

Do not drink cabbage juice if you have severe stomach acidity or irritated stomach symptoms. Therefore, sauerkraut is not healthy for patients with stomach ulcers, gastritis, or pancreatitis. Sauerkraut is harmful to hypertonicity in the body and people with kidney and liver diseases because the dish contains a large amount of salt. In this case, rinse cabbage with water before preparing the meal.

Stewed Sauerkraut

Stewed sauerkraut can be made either fresh and pickled. Sauerkraut can be stewed simply by simply boiling in water, but with the help of imagination it is possible to make a culinary masterpiece.

This recipe for stewed cabbages contains a lot of carrots, parsnips, and red peppers, creating an attractive variety of flavors and colors. Add boiled potatoes, or meat, sausages, ham, black plums, tomato paste, or just about anything your mind can "cook up."

Ingredients:

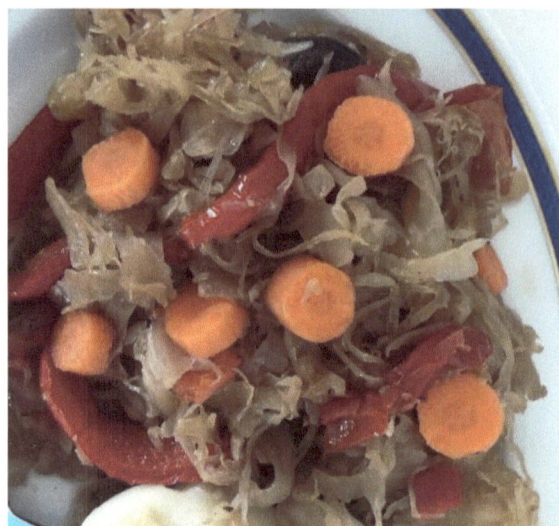

- 100 ml of Sunflower oil or other oil,
- 3 medium-sized onions,
- 1kg (2 oz) of pickled cabbage,
- 400g of carrots (3-4 carrots),
- 200g of parsnips, (2 pieces)
- 100g of red peppers (1 piece),
- 2 teaspoons of universal spices,
- 1 teaspoon of grounded black pepper,
- 350 ml of water,
- 2 teaspoons of cumin.

Preparation:

1. Slice the onions into small, semi-circular slices.
2. Add the sunflower oil to the frying pan, pour onions, and cook on low heat until the onions get a light golden color.
3. When the onions are fried, take them to a big pot of hot water, add washed, peeled and grated parsnips and carrots.
4. Stew the vegetables on low heat, stirring frequently.
5. Add the red pepper to the pot, mix all the contents together, and heat it for about 2-3 minutes.
6. Add spices. Adjust their amount according to your taste.
7. Add sauerkraut and mix everything well.
8. Water should be enough to cover the whole content of stewed vegetables. Cover the pot and cook for 40 minutes on low heat.
9. After 40 minutes, add the cumin. Check if the cabbage has already been softened. If so, serve hot with boiled potatoes.

Cauliflower Florets

Ingredients: (for four persons).
- 1 medium-sized cauliflower, about 50 gm
- ¼ cup butter 1 garlic clove,
- 2 eggs, hard boiled,
- ½ teaspoon of salt,
- ½ cup of grated cheese (Swiss, Jarlsberg, Parmesan, Pecorino, Gruyere or mix two varieties), and
- freshly ground pepper.

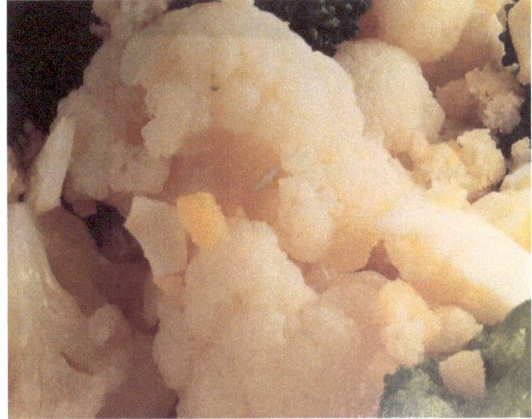

Preparation:
1. Cut the cauliflower, separate the florets and place them in a steamer over a pan of boiling water.
2. Steam for 5-7 minutes, until just tender.
3. Toss the steamed florets in butter and cheese mix and transfer to the main dish.
4. Finely chop the eggs and mix together with remaining ingredients.
5. Sprinkle the chopped egg mixture over the cooked florets. Serve warm.

Broccoli

Broccoli (Brassicaceae). Broccoli developed in Brussels and was brought to England in the mid eighteenth century and from there spread across Europe. It's believed that Italians brought it to America, where it became popular in the early 20th century.

In studies on the vegetable, scientists found a concentration of antioxidants in the florets, as well as a very high content of vitamin C and sulfolane. This composition guarantees the strong protection of the body, even from diseases such as cancer.

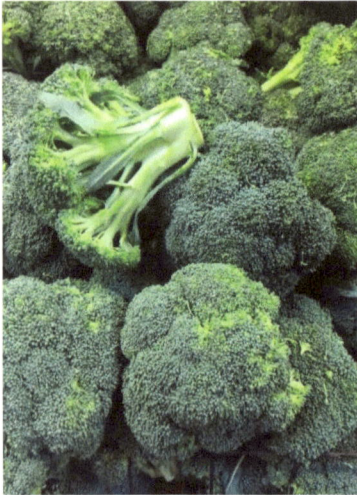

Preparation: It is very important that the broccolis are prepared in such a way as to avoid loss of useful nutrients. It is best to cook broccoli on a grill, or otherwise steam or cook it in small amounts of water for no more than three minutes as the flowers of broccoli must remain crisp. It is also advisable to cut the flowers with thin stems.

Frozen broccoli can last longer, but some of their beneficial ingredients disappear. The green flowers of the broccoli are suitable for adding to cabbage, while baked broccoli is suitable for meat, fish, and ground soups. Broccoli also goes well in cheese fondues, oriental dishes, pasta, and omelets.

What is Special about Broccoli

100 g broccoli contains 2.5 g carbohydrates, 3 g ballast materials, 0.2 g fat, and 3.5 g proteins. Broccoli is a vegetable that is rich in vitamins C, A, folic acid, nicotinic acid, riboflavin, thiamine, and B6 vitamins. In addition to vitamins, broccoli contains many micro-elements that are vital to our body: selenium, iron, calcium, copper, zinc, sodium, phosphorus, and magnesium, in addition to some very strong antioxidants; namely, alpha and beta-carotene, lutein, and zeaxanthin. Researchers have also found very important fatty acids for the human body in broccoli—omega-3 and omega-6. Like other cabbages, broccoli has the ability to reduce bad cholesterol in the body.

Benefits of Broccoli

Broccoli is recommended for those who are allergic to cow's milk to meet the calcium needs. It also has plenty of carotene, iron, vitamin C, and sodium; thus, this vegetable is suitable for those with an impaired kidney function. As they are easy to digest, they are suitable for those who are sick or are undergoing a period of fasting. Due to its low carbohydrate content, broccoli is suitable for diabetics.

Broccoli protects against gastric ulcers and intestinal ulcers caused by certain types of bacteria, boosting recovery time from ulcers. They also help digestion and prevent constipation. Broccoli cleans the body, helps to maintain a healthy body weight, and protects against osteoporosis.

If eaten regularly, Broccoli can reduce respiratory infections, inflammations, and allergies, so can help suppress asthma attacks. It will counter the effects of tobacco.

Broccoli reduces inflammatory processes in the body, and for people with a weak immunity, broccoli rebuilds the white blood cells, which effectively fighting the bacteria of various diseases. These anti-inflammatory properties improve the heart's circulation and help women with menstrual discomfort.

It has long been known that people eating a lot of vegetables and fruits often avoid oncological diseases. Broccoli should stand first on the list of healthy vegetables, and in this case, sulfolane helps in this fight against cancer.

Broccoli is not recommended to eat when …

If you are sick after eating broccoli then you should check your thyroid gland activity. It could be that you do not have enough iodine in your body, because that is the exact reaction the broccoli can provoke.

If broccoli becomes yellowed, they were probably stored for too long and spoiled. In this case they have lost valuable substances and their taste would be bitter. The leaves should be fresh and crispy.

Cooking with broccoli
In French cuisine, broccoli stalks are used as potatoes after peeling. The pulp under the skin is cut and placed in soups and stews. Most people throw away broccoli leaves without knowing that it is the most valuable part of broccoli as it contains a lot of selenium and it enhances the defensive forces of body. Peel the stalk and cut it into slices. Cook with the blossoms to keep the delicate taste. The stalks are good with nutritious salads. Popular additions to broccoli include adding a touch of spice, lemon juice, a little bit of garlic, grated nutmeg, and fried cedar nuts.

Recipe:

Warm Broccoli Salad

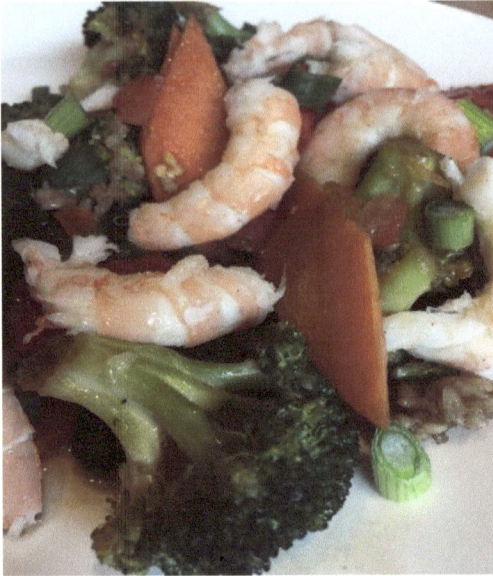

This vegetable can become the main ingredient in many salads and a balanced nutritional element.

Ingredients:
- 1kg (½ pound) broccoli,
- 2 tomatoes,
- 1 green pepper,
- ½ onion,
- 150g; (6-7) ready-made shrimps,
- sunflower oil for baking,
- olive oil for pouring on salad,
- a little pepper, a pinch of salt.

Preparation: Wash and chop the broccoli. Place broccoli in a steamer 3-4 minutes. Toss the broccoli in a bowl. Slice the tomatoes into cubes, the paprika in strips, and the onion in thin rings. Fry them in a frying pan for a few minutes and add shrimps. At the end of baking, mix everything with broccoli. Flavor with pepper and salt, and add a little olive oil.

Broccoli Salad with Dried Cranberries

Ingredients:
- 2 medium-sized broccoli heads,
- 2 medium-sized carrots,
- 2 hard sweet-sour apples,
- 100 g (½ cup) of dried cranberries,
- 50 g (2-3 tablespoons) of walnuts,
- salt,
- 200 ml yogurt without any additives.

Preparation: Rinse, cut the broccoli into small pieces or leave it in larger pieces if blanched in boiling water for several seconds. If you use the green stalk, cut it finely. Blush the cranberries with boiling water and drain.

Grate the carrots, slice the apples, and fry the nuts in a dry pan, and add salt to taste. Mix everything with yogurt or mayonnaise.

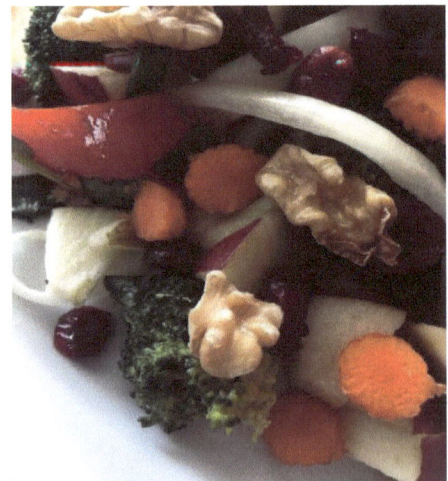

Beans

Beans (Phaseolus). A herbaceous shrub, or climbing plant, generally perennials. It is believed that beans originated in South America and were grown by Indians. In Europe, beans first began to be cultivated for food in the middle of 16th century in the Mediterranean region. There are approximately 150 known kinds of beans.

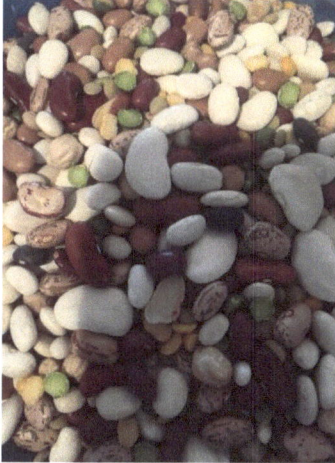

Bean Benefits

Beans contain a lot of iron, magnesium, potassium, copper, zinc, fiber, and protein. They are also very low in calories. There are plenty of starch and other carbohydrates and proteins, as well as almost all of the beneficial substances necessary for the body, such as vitamin C, B1, B2, B6, and PP. These legumes are rich in sulfur, which helps to cope with intestinal infections, rheumatism, and bronchial and skin diseases.

Because they contain a lot of iron, they are often included in the diet for the treatment of anemia, liver and kidney diseases, and diabetes.

Beans are not recommended to eat

Older people find that beans produce internal gas which can be uncomfortable. They are not recommended for eating in the presence of gout, nephritis, gastritis, ulcers, or pancreatitis.

Useful Tips

- Do not be afraid to buy canned beans. They are just as nutritious as untreated beans. Canned beans contain a lot of salt, which can be removed by running the beans for 1 minute under running water. When you buy canned beans, pay attention that the lid is not leveled. If it is, the beans will be spoiled.
- Before cooking, soak beans in water between 2 to 10 hours. Boil the beans without salt – add salt only at the end of cooking. Beans may take much longer to boil in heavy water than in soft water.
- To prevent the accumulation of gas, add mint to the dishes.
- If the beans have not completely ripened they may contain toxic substances; however, these substances break down with heat-treatment and become edible.

Cooked Bean Salad

Ingredients:
- 1 glass of white beans,
- 1 onion,
- 1 clove of garlic,
- 1 boiled egg,
- 2 potatoes,
- 4 carrots,
- 4 pickled cucumbers,
- 2 tablespoons of sour cream,
- 1 tablespoon of mayonnaise or olive oil,
- Salt and pepper to taste.

Preparation: Soak the beans in cold water overnight, then wash the beans again. Add 2 liters (2000 ml) of water to a large pot and boil the beans until they are soft, about 40 minutes. Add salt five minutes before finishing cooking. Drain and cool the beans. Cook clean and washed carrots and potatoes with the peel, and allow them to cool, then peel the potatoes. Finely chop the onion, garlic, pickled cucumbers and hard-boiled egg. Cut the chilled carrots and potatoes in small squares. Slice the vegetables and the egg before adding the sour cream, mayonnaise, and pepper. Mix the ingredients thoroughly in the bowl.

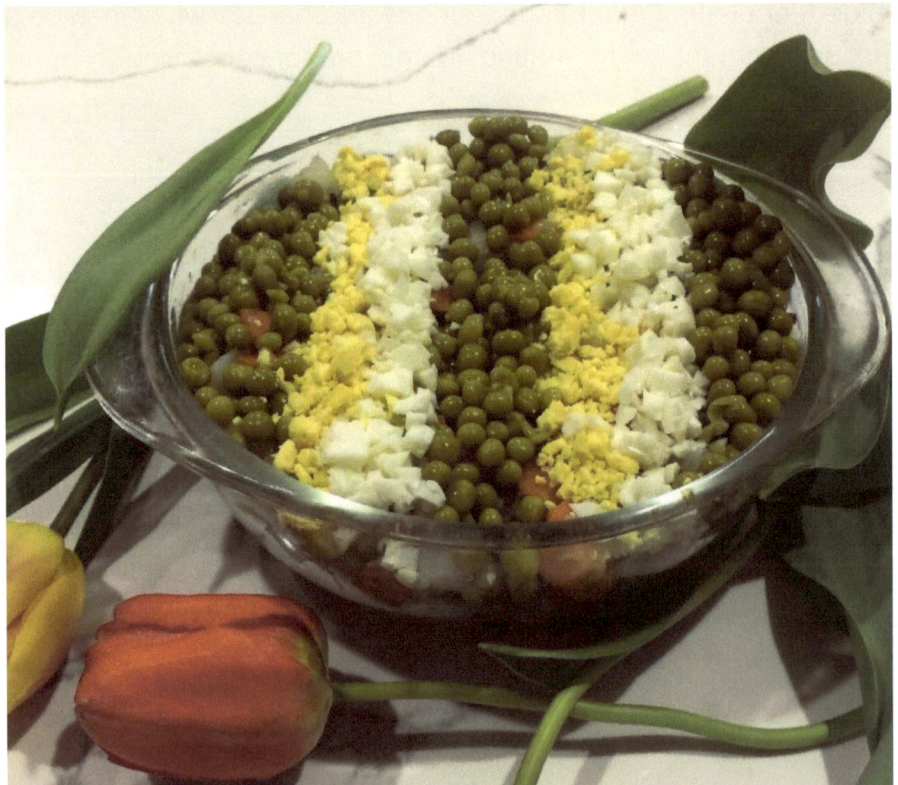

Spinach

Spinach (Spinacia oleracea) is an annual vegetable. The homeland of spinach was ancient Persia, and later imported to China. In Transcaucasia and Central Asia, some species of wild spinach are similar to cultivated spinach. In the Middle Ages the Arabs called spinach the "king of vegetables." During the Renaissance period, spinach spread through Europe, with monks becoming particularly fond of them, cultivating spinach on monastery farms. The culinary specialists of this period added ice, various creams, and sauces with spinach.

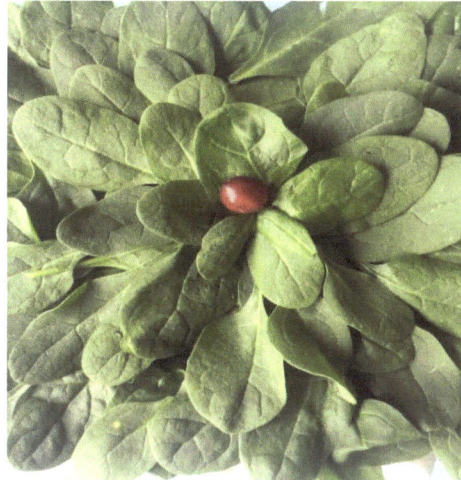

This plant is grown as a salad and likes fertilized, wet soil. Spinach is cold resistant and can be sown during autumn or spring. It is important to eat only fresh spinach, as harmful nitric acid salts develop as the cut leaves age.

The Benefits of Spinach

Spinach is used as a treatment by both traditional and folk medicine.

- Spinach is an easily digested vegetable rich in vitamins C, A, B1, B2, P, K, E D2, folic acid, and carotene. It contains iodine, mineral salts, iron, phosphorus, magnesium, sodium, and calcium. Spinach helps you to lose weight due its low calories content
- Spinach strengthens the immune system, helps to maintain healthy skin and hair, and positively affects the entire body.
- Not without a reason, the French people call the spinach a belly broom. Therefore, if you want to clean your body, eat spinach. Studies show that they remove waste from the body. Spinach juice calms gastric diseases.
- Swedish scientists claim that spinach embellishes the muscles, particularly for women who play sports. A daily intake of 300g spinach, even with minimal exercises, can increase the muscle mass.
- Spinach is believed to be beneficial to the gums. This is especially relevant for women, because they are at a greater risk of gum disease due to hormonal fluctuations during menopause and pregnancy.
- Spinach concoctions treat throat and respiratory diseases.
- Medical specialists say that spinach protects against anemia and tumors.
- Spinach is recommended for the treatment of tuberculosis, hypertension, anemia, nervous diseases, exhaustion, and diabetes mellitus.

Spinach is not recommended for eating if: you suffer from kidney inflammation, urinary bladder stones, gout, or diseases affecting the small intestine, liver, or gallbladder.

Pkhali, a snack with spinach and nuts

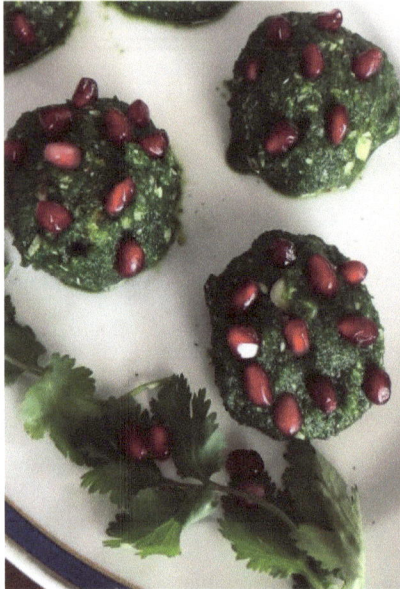

Pkhali is a Georgian Christmas dish, delightful in its green and red colors. This snack is quick and easy to prepare. To garnish the dish, sprinkle pomegranate seeds to create an artistic combination of beautiful colors.

Ingredients:

- 2 onions,
- 1 cup of finely chopped walnuts,
- ½ kg (1 pound) of spinach (fresh or frozen)
- 1 glass of pomegranate seeds.
- 1 teaspoon of parsley,
- 3 cloves of garlic,
- 1 teaspoon khmeli-suneli spice mix (if available),
- Various spices such as: a pinch of salt and pepper, a pinch of coriander (Coriandrum sativum)

Preparation:

1. Peel the onion and garlic
2. In a blender place walnuts, parsley, coriander, onions, garlic, salt and pepper and blend until very smooth.
3. Add washed and dried spinach and khmeli-suneli spices, and blend again.
4. Pour out the mixture and form dough-balls
5. Add the pomegranate seeds for decoration

Tomato

Tomato (Lycopersicon esculentum). Europeans first discovered tomatoes during their invasion of Mexico in the early 16th century. They initially called them *mala peruviana* (Peruvian apple), although the name changed to *tomate* from the Aztec word *tomatl*.

When the Spanish conquerors settled in Mexico (1519), their commander, Cortez, arranged the transportation of a shipment of tomatoes to Spain, a collection of yellow, white, orange, and red fruits. From Spain, tomatoes crossed the isthmus to Morocco where Italian sailors picked them up. These tomatoes were yellow and the Italians called them *pomodoro* (yellow golden apple), and later, known as *pomi del moro* (Moorish apples). By the end of the sixteenth century, the tomato became very popular in Italy and became a daily meal. Round, red tomatoes were first cultivated by the French naturalist Joseph Pitton de Tournefort in 1700, calling them *la pomme d 'amour,* "love apples." Fried tomatoes have long been adored by the Greeks and the Spanish.

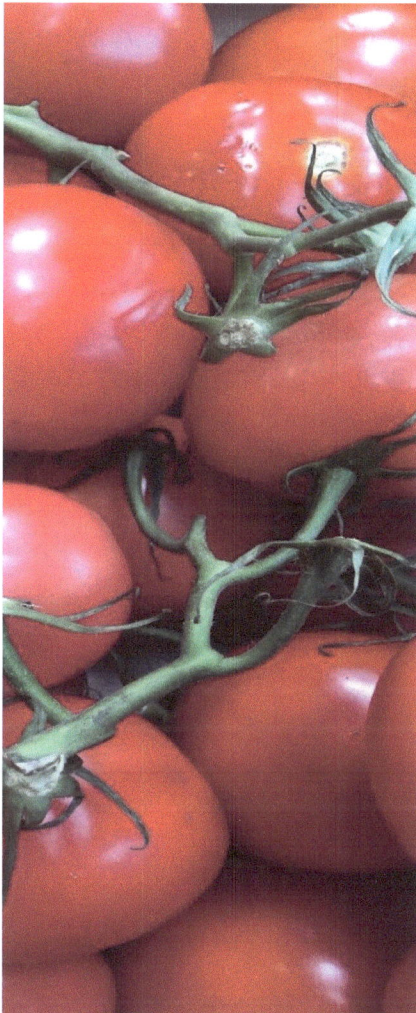

Until recently, many people believed that tomatoes were toxic plants, relating them to henbanes, tobacco, petunia, and potatoes. In America, the Puritans brought a negative attitude to tomato from England, listing tomatoes in the "Prohibited List," along with dances, songs, playing cards, and theater.

U.S. President Thomas Jefferson was the first to convince Americans that tomatoes were not toxic. In 1774, he cultivated several types of tomatoes in his garden in Virginia, serving them to guests, but the popularization of tomatoes still came slowly. In 1820, Robert Gibson Johnson consumed a basket of tomatoes on the steps of a courthouse in Salem, New Jersey. Two-thousand people gathered to see how Major Johnson could poison himself; however, this brave man did not die and lived until the age of 79.

Tomatoes and Health

Being both tasty and healthy, tomatoes serve as a valuable nutritional product. Tomatoes contain plenty of micro and macronutrients, excellent source of vitamins. Tomatoes contain all four major carotenoids: alpha and beta carotene, lutein and lycopene, which are thought to have the highest antioxidant activity of all the carotenoids. Metabolism of tomato carotenoids and their impact of human health has many health benefits, including lowering the risk of heart disease and cancer. Even tinned tomatoes maintain their vitamin C.

Tomatoes are recommended for people with anemia or heart weakness. If you have these problems, then you should eat an abundance of tomatoes. The fibers in tomatoes help to reduce the amount of sugar in the bloodstream, benefiting diabetics. 100g of tomatoes contain 1.2 gm fibers, which is useful in the treatment of constipation.

Tomatoes support skin elasticity, protect against harmful environmental effects, and protect the skin from ultraviolet rays.

If you wish to keep their rich and natural aroma never put tomatoes in the refrigerator; instead keep them in a cupboard and wash them just before preparation.

Recipe

Tomato Salad with Goat Cheese

If you do not have any delicious goat cheese, you can substitute Italian mozzarella or Greek feta.

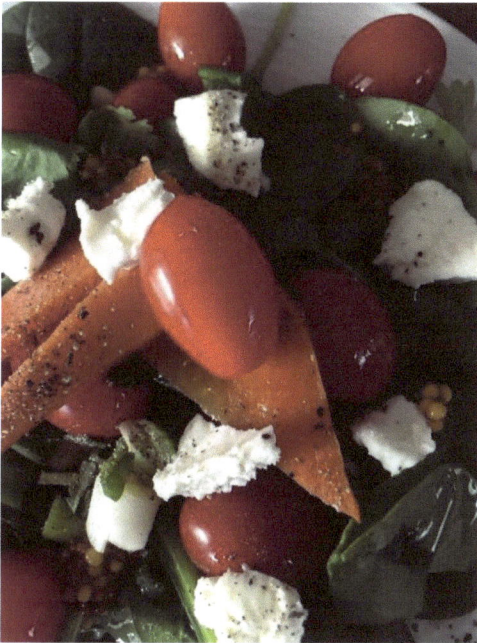

Ingredients:
- a mixture of various salads, about one cup per person
- Four large washed and sliced tomatoes, or, as in this picture, cherry or grape tomatoes.

Salad dressing:
- 1 garlic clove minced,
- 1 teaspoon of mustard,
- juice from 2 lemons,
- six teaspoons of extra-virgin olive oil,
- 1.5 oz of goat cheese,
- kosher salt,
- freshly ground black pepper,
- four teaspoons of parsley or basil (chop fresh before serving to the table.)

Preparation:
1. Put a layer of greens onto separate plates with some sliced tomatoes on top. Add salt to the mixture.
2. Mix the dressing components.
3. Crush the cheese on the tomatoes.
4. Add salt and pepper to taste.
5. Apply the dressing and add chopped parsley.
6. Serve with a slice of French white bread.

Red Beets

Beetroot is a biennial vegetable of the Amaranthaceae family of the beetroot (beta) tribe, which derives from self-grown beetroot. Beetroots were domesticated in the Mediterranean region in the 11th-millennium B.C. and later spread throughout Mesopotamia and China. The root is used for food, as well as fresh leaves and cuttings. Beetroots are often incorporated into soups and salads. By the times of ancient Greece and Rome, they were consumed both as food and as a medicine. Even then, this vegetable was recognized as a source of health and longevity.

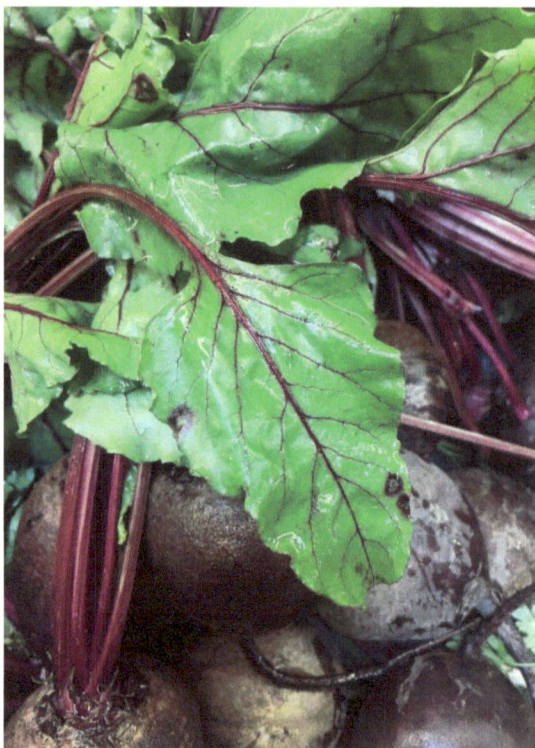

Beetroot and their Health Benefits

Beetroot is rich in a number of minerals, such as betaine, and a significant amount of vitamins, including P (flavonoids), B complex, and vitamin C, which helps the immune system. Beetroot leaves are rich in vitamin A.

Beetroot strengthens the hemoglobin levels, helping prevent anemia thereby helping to rebuild strength after exhaustion. Cooked beetroots build strong gums and help improve digestion. The high levels of folic acid in beetroot give a glow and elasticity to one's skin. Beetroot has a positive effect on the condition of bones and arteries. By facilitating the removal of toxins from the body, it reduces the risk of the formation of malignant tumors. On top of this, it cleanses the kidneys and blood, reduces the acidity of the body, and protects against radioactive and heavy metals.

Even cooked beetroots save useful substances and minerals. **If you have a sensitive stomach or a high acidity, drink beetroot juice carefully, perhaps diluting it with other juices.**

Recipe:

Summer Cold Beetroot Soup with Yogurt

This cold, refreshing soup is great during hot summer periods. It is easy to prepare and nourishing. The soup is made with yogurt that contains a lot of protein, thereby eliminating the need for meat bouillon, so you can even eat it without a main dish of fish or meat. Red beetroot has a lot of fiber, and its bright color rivets the attention. This dish can be eaten as a dinner or supper meal.

Ingredients:
- 2 medium-sized beetroots,
- 2 cups of yogurt (without additives),
- 2 cups of buttermilk,
- ½ cup of boiled cold water,
- shallots or simple garlic cloves,
- 2 hard-boiled eggs,
- 2 green cucumbers,
- 1 tablespoon of dill,
- a little parsley, and
- 2 fresh potatoes.

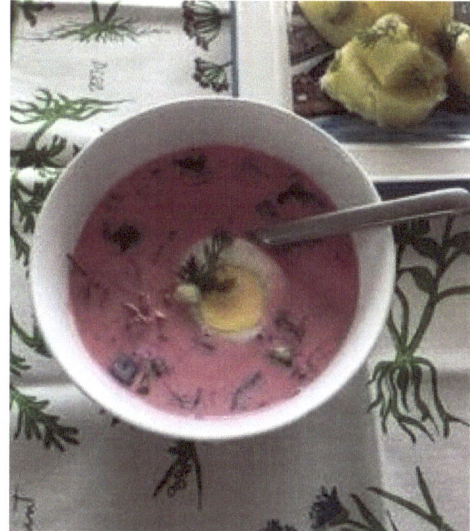

Preparation: Cook the beetroots until they are softened, then peel them and slice or grate with a beetroot grater. Peel and finely chop the garlic, cucumber, hard-fried eggs, spring onions, and dills. Put it in a bowl and pour 2 cups of yogurt over the mixture and add 2 cups of buttermilk, and a ½ cup of cold boiled water. Spread the chopped parsley and dill over the cold beetroot and serve in bowls with freshly cooked or fried potatoes.

Zucchini

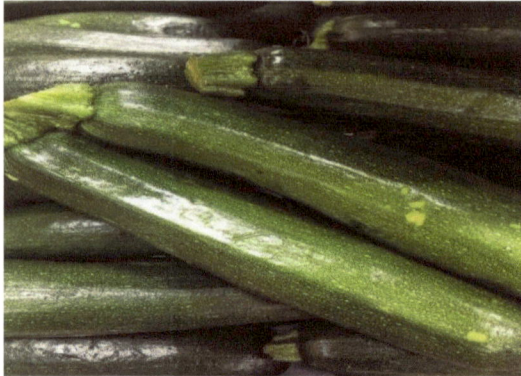

Zucchini (Cucurbita pepo). Zucchini originated as a cucumber hybrid on the sunny Mexican coast. It came to Europe in the 16th century and spread widely, now found throughout the world. The current vegetable we call zucchini was developed in Italy in the 19th century.

The zucchini grows very fast and must be supervised so that it does not overgrow. Young zucchini is the most valuable type and should be harvested at 15 - 30 centimeters in length. The longer a zucchini stays on the vine, the more its taste decreases, and it can grow up to a meter in length.

Health Benefits of Zucchini

- 100g of the zucchini contains 15 calories without any cholesterol.
- Zucchini is a vegetable that contains a lot of minerals, pectins, carotenes, carbohydrates, vitamins, and mild fibers, with a low sugar content. The best zucchinis are those that are small and greenish white in color, as these contain more minerals and useful substances
- Zucchini increases the physical and mental capacity for work, strengthens the nerves and brain, and activates protein synthesis in each cell.
- Zucchini stimulates the excretion of water from the body, aids weight loss, eliminates intestinal toxins, and activates peristalsis; therefore, it is very healthy for the intestines.
- Zucchini regulates the heart rate and blood pressure, removes toxic substances, strengthens the immune system, and stimulates metabolism.
- The zucchini is commonly used in cosmetics since it is suitable for face masks, especially those made for dry and sensitive skin, however, the most effective mask is for foot skin. Apply the thinly cut zucchini to the hardened skin of the soles and wrap the sole with a sterile gauze or a clean cloth. Keep it wrapped for 30 minutes, before washing it and applying cream.

Cooking with zucchini

You can prepare zucchini in many different ways, such as roasted or stuffed (green zucchinis are rarely used like this), in salads and sauces, with fried pancakes or in potato-based dishes such as kugel, and even in jams and compotes. If you want to make delicious jam, it is best to use acidic fruit because the zucchini is not sour at all. For example, tinned pineapple juice with chopped zucchini is a tasty dessert.

If you stew zucchini, add a little bit of oil to ensure that the fat-soluble pro-vitamin A is optimally absorbed into the body. You can also flavor aromatic zucchini dishes with various herbs, such as oregano, tarragon, and lemon balm.

Zucchini suits well with other vegetables, namely red peppers, tomatoes, onions, and garlic.

Zucchini Pancakes

Ingredients:
- 2 small zucchinis,
- 2 eggs,
- 1 onion,
- 8 tablespoons flour,
- 20 g (1 tablespoon) of dill,
- ½ cup of oil,
- a pinch of salt,
- black pepper.

Preparation:
1. Grate zucchinis with a large grater. Peel and chop finely onions and dill.
2. Put the eggs in the grated zucchini, pour flour, onions, and dill, add salt and pepper, and mix well.
3. Bake in well-heated oil. Put a large spoon of dough and make a pancake. Fry on both sides until they become beautifully crisp. Be careful not to break the pancakes. Serve hot.
Tip: Sour cream and garlic sauce goes deliciously with these pancakes. Press a slice of garlic into a glass of sour cream, add salt and sliced dill, and mix well.

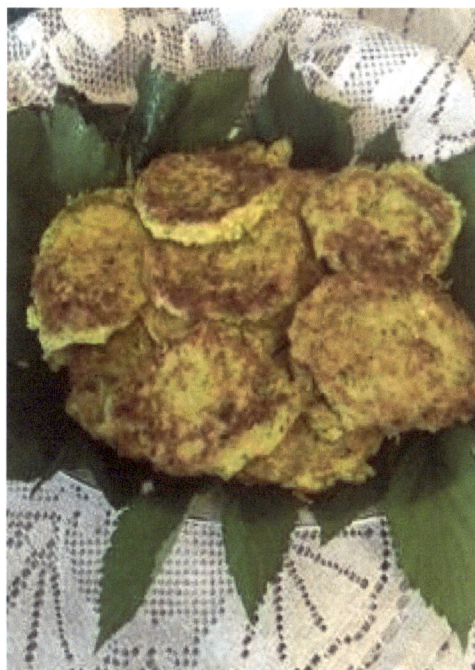

Sweet Potatoes

The sweet potato is also known as the Batatas (Ipomoea batatas). This plant belongs to the morning glory family, whose tubers are used for food. The sweet potato is widely used across the globe, and particularly in the Far East, African, and South East Asian cuisines. The people from these regions typically eat sweet potatoes either cooked or fried, or with cakes and as an ingredient in other sweet dishes. The sweet potato originated in South America. Due to the abundance of accumulated nutrients, it is considered one of the most useful vegetables in the world. Sweet potatoes have more nutrients than simple potatoes.

One potato contains more than 100% of the required amount of vitamin A, 37% of vitamin C, 16% of vitamin B6, 10% of vitamin B5, 15% of potassium, and 28% of manganese. It also contains calcium, iron, magnesium, phosphorus, and other minerals, as well as vitamins B1, E, B2, and B9. In addition, the potato is a great source of carotene, a strong antioxidant.

Health Benefits of Sweet Potatoes

Sweet potatoes regulate the blood sugar in the body. The dietary fiber present in sweet potatoes is useful for diabetics. Sweet potato strengthens the immune system due to its antioxidant nutrients, boosts memory, reduces inflammation, improves digestion, and improves eyesight.

Do not consume sweet potatoes if you suffer from kidney disorders because sweet potatoes contain high levels of potassium.

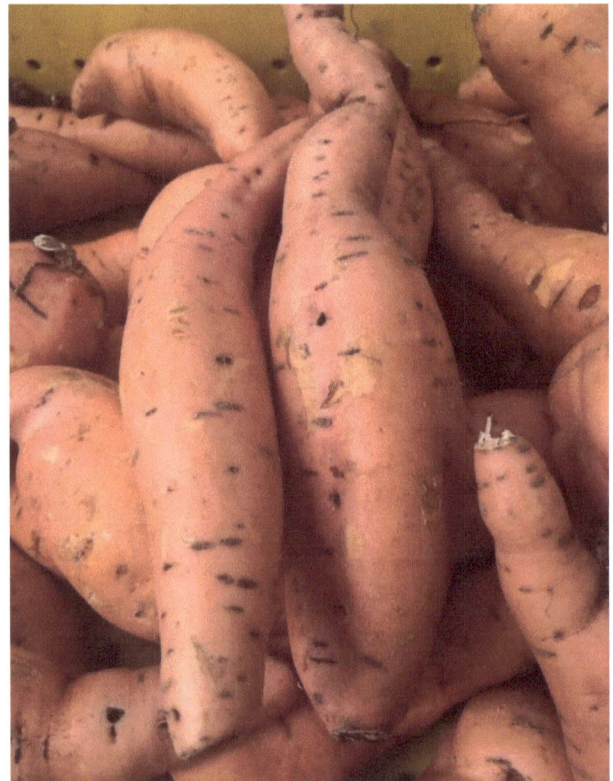

Recipe:

This wonderful sweet potato recipe tastes like a dessert. This side dish is welcome at any meal and will make your house smell like an aromatic dream and provide a dish rich in vitamins and fiber. Perfect for every time of the year as well as the holidays.

Sweet Potatoes with Apples and Cinnamon

Ingredients:
- 3 sweet potatoes
- 4 apples
- 1 teaspoon ground cinnamon
- 1/2 cup orange juice
- 1/4 cup brown sugar

Preparation: Preheat oven to 350 degrees F (175 Degrees C).
Wash, peel and cut sweet potatoes in thin rounds.
Peel, core, and cut apples into rings or thin slices.
In a small bowl, mix brown sugar and cinnamon.
In a casserole dish, layer the sweet potatoes and apples.
Pour orange juice over the top.
Sprinkle brown sugar over potatoes and apples and in between every layer. (If apples are sweet, there's no need to add sugar, just cinnamon).
Bake covered in the preheated oven for 35-45 minutes or until potatoes and apples become tender.

Pumpkin

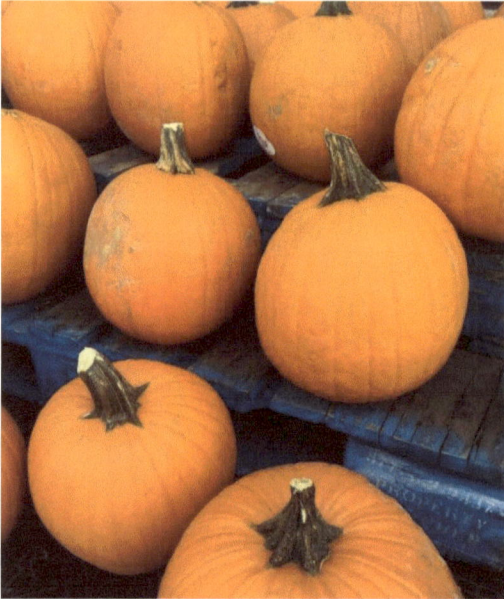

Pumpkin (Cucurbita). Pumpkins are widespread in North America, of which there are many different types. Normally, the pumpkin is a light orange or yellow color.

100 g of pumpkin amounts to only 26 calories. Pumpkins do not contain cholesterol.

Health Benefit of Pumpkin

The pumpkin is an excellent antioxidant as it is one of the best sources of carotene, which thus lends it its orange color. Carotene turns into vitamin A in the body, and the pumpkin is also a great source of other nutrients, vitamins, and minerals.

The pumpkin improves mood, sleep, digestion, appetite, and vision, and it maintains heart health. Pumpkin seeds are rich in magnesium, iron, proteins, and zinc, which help to keep healthy strong bones and a low blood pressure. When eating pumpkin seeds, it is best to buy them prepared without salt.

Pumpkin Cake

Ingredients:
- 2 1/4 cups of all-purpose flour, (400g.)
- 1 teaspoon of baking soda
- 1 teaspoon of vanilla
- 1 teaspoon of cinnamon
- pinch of salt
- ½ (100g) to 1 cup (per taste) of brown sugar
- 1¾ cups unsweetened preserved pumpkin purée (best organic), or mashed pumpkin
- 2 eggs
- ½ cup of oil or dissolved butter (100g)
- 1 cup dried or fresh cranberries.

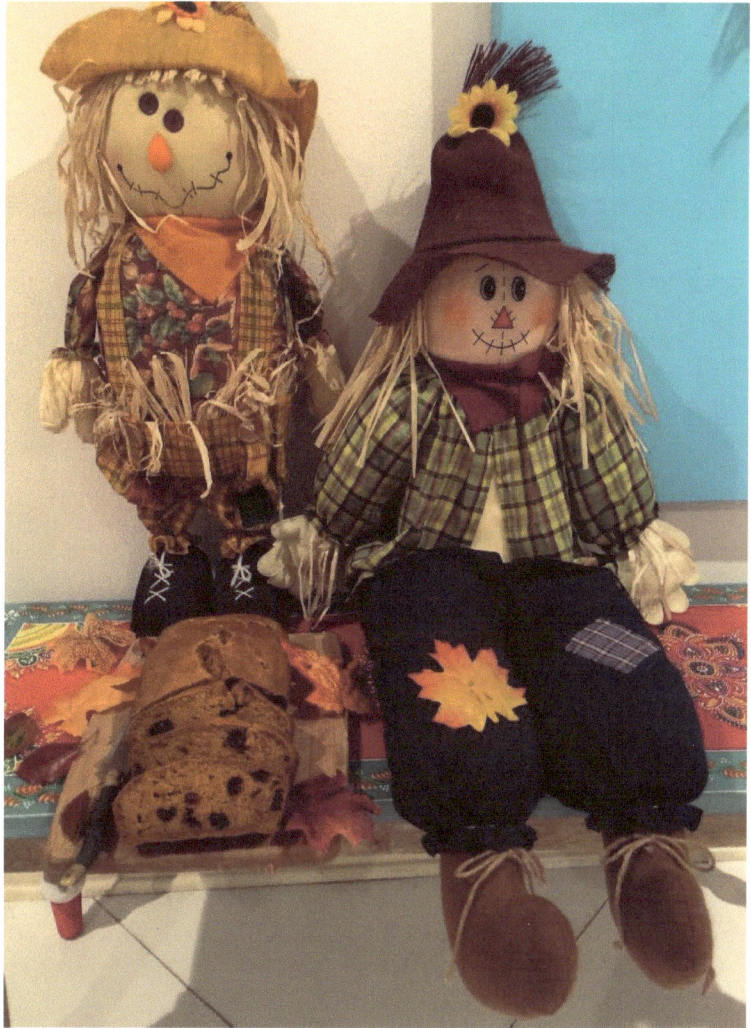

Preparation: Preheat oven to 350 degrees F (175 C), grease a pan with butter. Mix flour with soda, cinnamon and salt in a bowl. In another bowl, mix the eggs with sugar, pour oil or butter, vanilla, and add pumpkin and cranberries. Mix well until smooth. Slowly beat flour mixture into pumpkin until consistency is smooth. Pour into prepared cake pan.

Bake in the preheated oven until a toothpick inserted in the center of the cake comes out clean, about 30-40 minutes.

Cool the cake before cutting it.

Onions

Garden onion (Allium cepa). A long time ago, this plant spread throughout Egypt, Italy, and Greece, however, the homeland of the garden onion is Central Asia. The shepherds of Afghanistan, Iran, and Turkmenistan wandered through the mountain paths and were the first ones to recognize this plant.

The medicinal properties of onions were known in the ancient Eastern countries where the saying, "Onion, when you touch me, any illness passes," was commonplace.

Onions have a sharp smell and taste due to irritating mucous quercetin glycosides.

They contain helpful digestive enzymes and the vitamins C, B1, B2, PP (Niacin), as well as carotenoids, saccharides, inulin, amino acids, pectins, microelements, and other substances.

Onion plants can grow up to 60cm high. Both the lower and upper part of the onion is edible, and the upper green part of the onion is known as the Spring Onion.

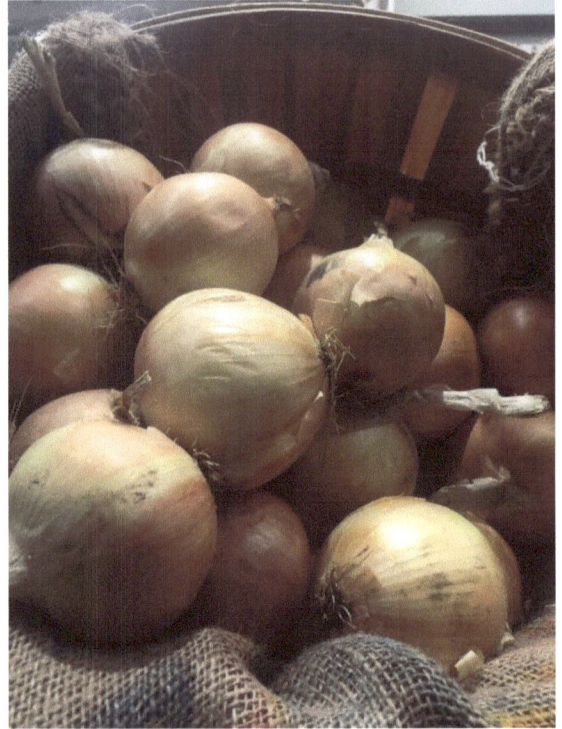

Onion Healing Properties

1. Onions reduce blood pressure, cholesterol levels, stimulate blood circulation, and protect against colds. For atherosclerosis, it is advisable to make a mixture of onion juice and honey in equal parts. Drink this mixture 1 teaspoon 3-4 times a day.
2. To improve overall body condition, eat 15-100 g of stewed, steamed, oven cooked, or dried onions 1-2 times a day, 15 minutes before eating. Course duration: 2-3 weeks
3. To strengthen the body or improve impaired hearing or sight, drink fresh onion juice evenly mixed with 1 teaspoon of honey 3-4 times a day, and before eating in the morning.
4. For intestinal diseases it is advisable to take 1 teaspoon of onion juice before eating.
5. For insect stings, grease the spot with onion juice. The pain will quickly disappear.
6. For hair loss or scalp problems, scrub the scalp with fresh onion juice twice a week.
7. Active onion ingredients, such as quercetin, help to protect against colds and flu.

8. To prevent the spread and accumulation of microbes through the air, cut a slice of onion and put it near the bed at night.
9. When you have a stuffy nose, fold a few pieces of mashed onion in a gauze and hold this under your nose.
10. At the first signs of cold and flu, moisten a gauze or cloth with onion juice and place it in the nostrils for 10-15 minutes three times a day.

The best way to use the onion is in its fresh and uncooked form, adding it to salads, sandwiches, soups, garnishes, sauces, and other dishes.

Do not use onions if you suffer from acute gastric, intestinal, kidney, or liver problems, or if you have duodenal ulcers.

1. **Green Onion Salad**

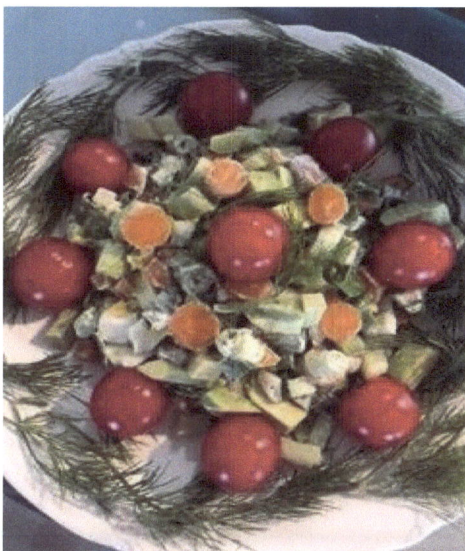

Ingredients:
- 200g (one handful) spring onions,
- 2 eggs,
- 3 tablespoons of sour cream or olive oil,
- ½ tsp lemon juice,
- 2 cloves garlic,
- 2 tomatoes (or baby plum tomatoes),
- 2 small cucumbers,
- 1 cooked carrot,
- 1 teaspoon of dill,
- 1 avocado,
- 1 slice pineapple,
- a pinch of salt and pepper.

Preparation: Chop boiled eggs with sliced spring onions, cucumbers, boiled carrot and crushed garlic. Add sliced dill, spices, lemon juice, and the sour cream, or oil. Mix thoroughly and place in the salad bowl. Sprinkle the surface with chopped avocado and tomato slices or add baby plum tomatoes.

2. French Onion Soup

Onions have always been an irreplaceable part of French cuisine. A popular legend tells us that this soup was prepared for the first time by King Louis XV when he came to a hunter's house late one evening and the cook there was caught unprepared for the king's reception. Thus, the King himself tried to prepare something tasty but could find nothing more than butter, champagne, and onions. From this point forward, French Onion Soup became a huge success.

The most important thing while preparing this soup is patience, so as to get the perfect flavor and aroma.

Ingredients: (4-6 portions).
- 4 big onions,
- 1 stick of unsalted butter, or ½ cup of sunflower oil, or olive oil,
- 2 teaspoons of all-purpose flour,
- 6-7 cups (1.5-1.8 liters) of homemade beef broth (can be chicken, vegetables, mushroom broth),
- 100-200 ml of dry white wine or 2-3 tablespoons of brandy,
- Kosher salt and ground black pepper,
- 2 bay leaves to taste,
- a French baguette (if a French baguette is left for a long time and dried in the kitchen it is perfect to prepare it for use as a sippet.)
- fermented cheese (grated Gruyere is the best),
- several twigs of thyme.

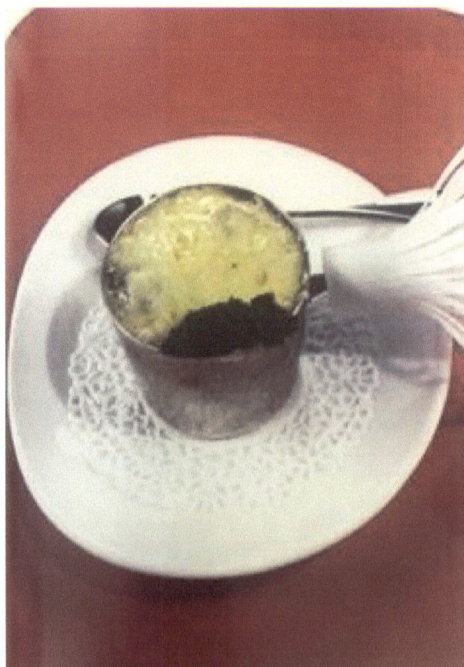

Preparation: Slice the onion into thin slices, add sunflower oil to the pan and cook them for about 30 minutes until the onions get a yellowish shade - caramelized. When baked onions are fully caramelized, add 2 teaspoons of flour, stir and fry for 1 minute, then add 2 tablespoons of broth. Mix it again and pour it into a saucepan. Add 100-200 ml wine. When the soup boils, add spices, cover, and cook on a low heat and simmer for about 35 minutes. When cooking, mix occasionally. If you do not use wine, 2-3 tablespoons of brandy can be added at the end of cooking. Taste the soup to know whether there are enough spices.

Prepare the sippets. Cut 1 slice of baguette for a portion and sprinkle it with grated cheese, or put a thin slice of cheese on a baguette. Place the sippets with cheese on the baking tray and let them cook in the heated oven for several minutes until the cheese melts. For each serving, pour hot onion soup into bowls and place the prepared sippets with melted cheese on the top of the bowl. Decorate with thyme twigs. The onion soup must be served hot.

If you do not have an oven, put the prepared sippets in a large ceramic frying pan, cover them with a lid and heat until the cheese melts and the bottom of the sippet is baked. You do not need to fry sippets, just put them at the bottom of the bowl and pour a hot soup over them—the cheese will melt from the heat of the soup and the sippets themselves become softer. This soup is best eaten with a spoon, and by taking a slice of baguette with melted cheese.

Onion Peels

We often throw away onion peels without even knowing what benefits they can give us. Onion peels contain the vitamins C, E, PP, and B. They also contain potassium, calcium, magnesium, manganese, copper, zinc, chromium, aluminum, selenium, nickel, lead, boron, and iron.

1. Their decoction and infusion are effective helpers against microbes, stimulate bile secretion, help the internal organs, and help to clear one's throat
2. Many of our grandmothers washed their hair only with onion-peel water. They boiled onion peels for 10 minutes, cooled them, and then used that water to wash their hair. If we did this, our hair would be beautiful, shiny, and would not fall out.
3. Onion peels improve heart function, eliminate the excess of sodium and chlorine from the body, help to clear one's throat, facilitate defecation, and improve biliary excretion.
4. Folk medicine advises you to drink onion peel tea if you suffer from cramps or hypertonia, while onion peels additionally improve the cardiovascular system, have urine flow stimulation properties, and strengthen blood vessels by helping them to be more elastic.
5. Onion peels are host to a magic substance—quercetin—which not only contains anti-flu, anti-allergic, and antimicrobial properties, but it also protects against cramps, reduces blood pressure, improves kidney and brain performance, and helps against sclerosis.
6. In the case of a stroke, it is advisable to rub the paralyzed limb with onion tincture twice a day.

7. To restore the viability of the whole organism, drink the onion-peel water with lemon juice.
8. Itchy skin or dermatitis can be healed if you place a bandage soaked in the onion peel water on the inflamed area for 10 minutes twice daily.

Grind the onion peels with a coffee-mill and store tightly closed in a glass container. A useful and great flavor tea can be made with one teaspoon of ground onion peels. The tea will have a pink shade, and a teaspoon of ground ginger with ground lemon and a teaspoon of honey give it an extra kick.

To create a tincture, mix 3 tablespoons of crushed onion peels with 300 ml of water and boil for 10 minutes. Cool at room temperature, filter out the peels, and add the juice of 2 lemons. It is advisable to take a ⅓ of a glass 3 times a day, 1 hour before the start of a meal for 14 to 21 days.

Since the onion peels have a very positive effect on the kidneys, it is useful to use an unpeeled, well-washed onion in the preparation of the dishes. When the food is cooked, the onion can be removed and thrown away. A bouillon prepared with an unpeeled onion will be golden and aromatic, look delicious, and find many uses during cooking.

A healing ointment of onion peels is suitable for the treatment of dandruff, nail fungus, furunculus, dermatitis, and acne. To prepare the healing ointment, finely chop the onion peels until they become a powder and mix with either baby cream, medical Vaseline, or butter at a ratio of 2:3 or 1:3. Store the ointment in a dark glass vial in a refrigerator. Regular application to problematic skin spots can lead to full healing.

Onion Peel Tincture for Nail Fungus Treatment:
Pour ½ l of vodka over 8 tablespoons of onion peels, and after 10 days apply the filtered tincture to fungus spots 3-4 times a day. It is advisable to continue this procedure for 7-10 days.

Onion peel water: Adding onion peels to regular tap water instills it with wonderful healing properties. Simply submerge 2-3 tablespoons of onion peels in 3 liters of tap water and store in natural light. Onion peel water destroys the pathogenic microflora in the soil, feeds it with microelements, revitalizes poor plants and gives them vitality. The color of cucumber leaves recovers if you use onion peel water for the yellowing cucumbers, causing the plant to grow more heavily and produce new offspring.

Lastly, to produce beautifully brown Easter eggs, wrap the eggs in onion peels and a gauze and add to boiling water for 5 minutes.

Leeks

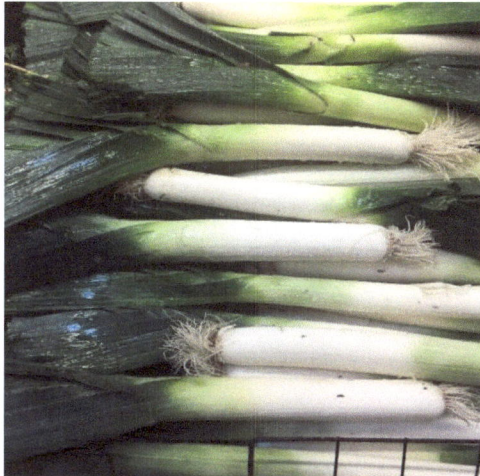

Leek (Allium porrum). Leeks come from Mediterranean countries and are particularly popular in England and France. This is both a biennial and a perennial plant, cultivating up to 50-100 cm stems, ending with a large flower ball-shaped head. They have a bitter odor and taste, although the heads of the leeks are sweeter than onion heads. It is advisable to eat the lower part of the stems of the leeks and their young and broad leaves. The old leaves are yellow and cannot be eaten.

Leek Healing Properties

The leeks are rich in vitamins C, B2, E, PP, and carotene. They promote urinary excretion, improve the functioning of liver and gallbladder, and improve appetite. The leeks regulate the functioning of the stomach and intestine.

Laxative: Cut 100 g of crushed leeks, pour a ½ cup of boiling water, boil for 3 minutes, and then filter the decoction. The decoction has a slight laxative effect.

Broths, vegetable soups, meat, and fish dishes may be flavored with leeks. They have low calories and are very nutritious. If you want to lose a bit of weight, leek soup on a slimming day will bring good results.

Eat leeks when you are hungry for breakfast, lunch, and dinner. Leeks have a sweet taste, and you can further enhance their flavor by spraying them with olive oil and lemon juice and add salt and pepper. This will be a weekend ration until Sunday dinner. After this, you can eat a 120-170 g piece of meat or fish with some stewed vegetables and some fruits.

You can mix them with vegetables, carrots, celery, or cauliflower. You can also boil or stew them and add a sliced and boiled egg to the soup.

Magic Leek Soup (Broth)

Ingredients:
- 1 kg of leeks.

Preparation: Clean the leeks and wash them so as not to leave sand or dirt. Cut away the dark green ends, leaving only the white stems and light greenery. Put the leeks into a large pot, cover them with water, and boil. Reduce the heat for 20-30 minutes and cook without covering the lid. Filter the broth into a separate container and put the heated leeks into a bowl.

Garlic

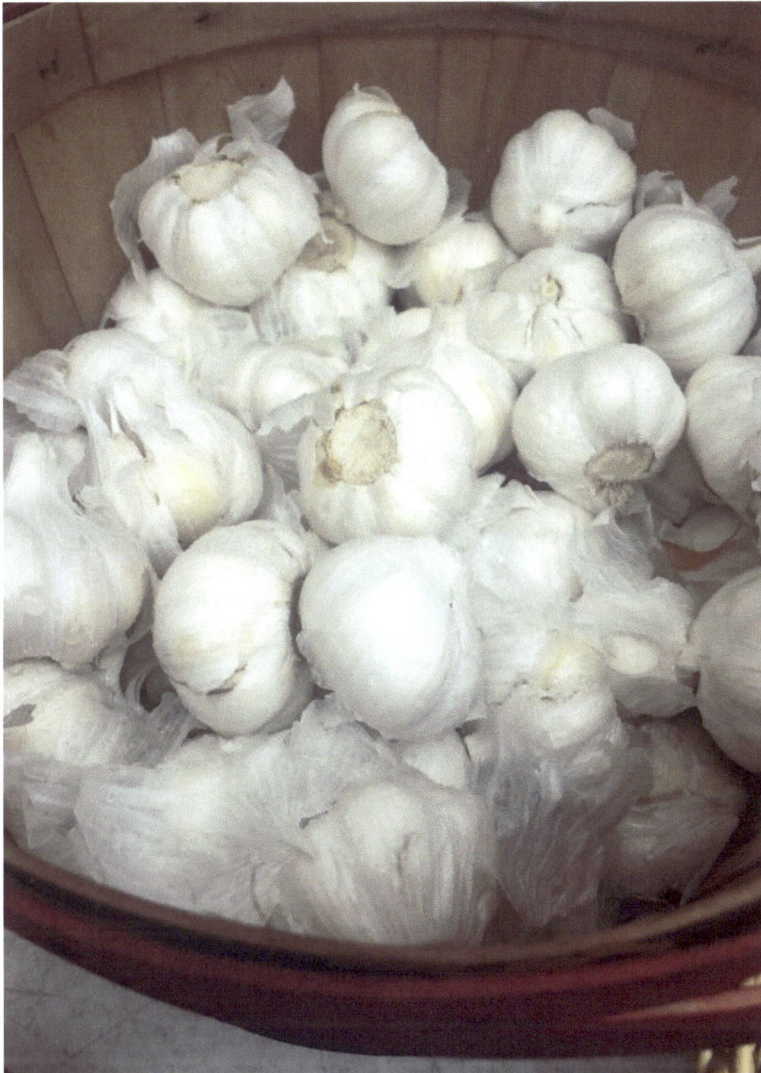

Garlic (Allium sativum) is a strong antibiotic. The ancient Egyptians, Greeks, and Romans considered garlic as a universal means of improving the body.

Garlic is a major ingredient in Indian cuisine. Garlic has been grown in Asia from immemorial times. The Italians, Greeks, Spanish, Jews, and French do not imagine food without garlic. It is said that a mixture of garlic, onions, and radishes was given to the builders of the pyramids. Garlic was a necessary entree to the gladiator's diet. Pythagoras called garlic "The king of spices," and the famous physician Avicenna knew thousands of recipes with garlic.

Garlic is rich in iodine, salt, and numerous vitamins and etheric oils.

Health Benefits of Garlic

1. An active ingredient of garlic is called allicin. It is a powerful antibiotic that inhibits harmful bacteria from growing and multiplying in our bodies.
2. Garlic slows the progression of cancer cells.
3. Garlic reduces decay processes in the intestine, increases the functioning of gastric and small intestines, and promotes cardiovascular activity.
4. Both the active substances of garlic and lemon cleanse the body effectively,
5. Garlic improves the skin's appearance, leaving it brighter, smoother, and more elastic.

6. Garlic also cures acne and pigmentation spots and improves mood, reduces fatigue, strengthens immunity, and reduces blood pressure.
7. Garlic is known as a remedy for intestinal parasites.
8. When a flu virus is spreading around your home or workplace, eat a few cloves of garlic daily with one tablespoon of apple jam (so as not to irritate the stomach). This will strengthen your immunity.

If you bought too much garlic, split it into slices, peel, and store them in a bowl of olive oil. Garlic will stay fresh for several months in the refrigerator, and the oil can be used for salad dressings.

Folk Recipe to Cleanse Blood Vessels

Honey, lemon, and garlic syrup. It is said that this syrup dissolves cholesterol plaques.
Ingredients:
- six large lemons
- 350 ml of liquid honey. The best honey comes from lime or field plants
- four garlic heads.

Preparation: wash the lemons well (to remove the remaining pesticides after spraying), then soak in a soda and water solution for 15-20 minutes. Cut and peel the garlic. Mix everything in an electric blender. Pour honey in the mass. Mix the syrup with a wooden spoon, pour it into a jar, shake well, and store in a dark place for 10 days. After 10 days, use 1 tablespoon of this syrup, dilute it with a glass of boiled warm water, and drink it each morning before eating, and again in the evening before bedtime. Keep this syrup in the refrigerator.

Blood cleaning with garlic and wine.
Ingredients:
- 12 garlic cloves,
- 3 red wine glasses.

Preparation: Cut each garlic clove into 4 parts, mix with red wine and pour into a jar. Close the jar and place it on the windowsill to ferment for about two weeks. Each day, shake the jar well. After two weeks, filter the mixture, which will have become a type of brandy, and pour it into a dark bottle. Drink 1 tablespoon three times a day. Course duration: 30 days.

Blood cleaning with garlic and vodka.
Ingredients:
- 100g of (30 ounces) of crushed garlic,
- 150 ml. vodka.

Preparation: Crushed garlic is mixed with 150 ml vodka in a bottle. Keep it tightly closed and store in a dark place for 10 days. To consume, shake well, percolate, and take 20 drops (preferably with milk) 2-3 times a day for 30 minutes before eating.

Garlic butter—an effective antimicrobial agent.
Preparation: Mix 5 cloves of crushed garlic with 100g (30 ounces) of butter and apply on bread or flavor with mashed potatoes.

Garlic and Lemon
Ingredients
- 2 peeled and crushed garlic heads,
- 2 washed and ground lemons with peel.

Preparation: Mix these components and place them in a tightly closed jar and keep in the refrigerator. Take 1 teaspoon 3 times a day for 30 minutes before a meal.

Garlic, Honey, and Lemon
Mix 1 liter of honey with 10 washed and ground lemons with peel and 10 peeled and ground garlic heads. Place all of the ingredients in a jar and close it tightly. After one week, use 3 teaspoons once a day. Each teaspoon of this mixture is chewed or sucked until finally swallowed. The amount of such a mixture is sufficient for 2 months.

Garlic should not be used if you suffer from epilepsy or kidney, stomach, or urinary tract diseases, or if you are pregnant.

You can remove the odor of the garlic by drinking warm milk or chewing coffee beans.

Carrot

Carrot (Daucus sativus). Carrot is one of the oldest widespread vegetables, consumed for more than 4000 years. It is believed they originated from wild carrots grown in Iran and Afghanistan. Nowadays, the common edible carrots come from Europe. They traveled from Europe to America, Australia, and New Zealand. Ancient Roman writers called the carrot the queen of the garden.

Carrots contain a lot of carotene, which then turns into vitamin A in the body, needed for the eyes and the body. Vitamin A also benefits the skin and mucous membranes. Carrots are rich in protein, flavonoids, essential oils, and minerals: cobalt, potassium, iron, copper, phosphorus, iodine, vitamins B1, B2, B6, C, E, K, and others. The best way to eat carrots is fresh to best preserve their vitamins and fiber. They have low calories (100g = 41 calories). There is no cholesterol. They're perfect for diets.

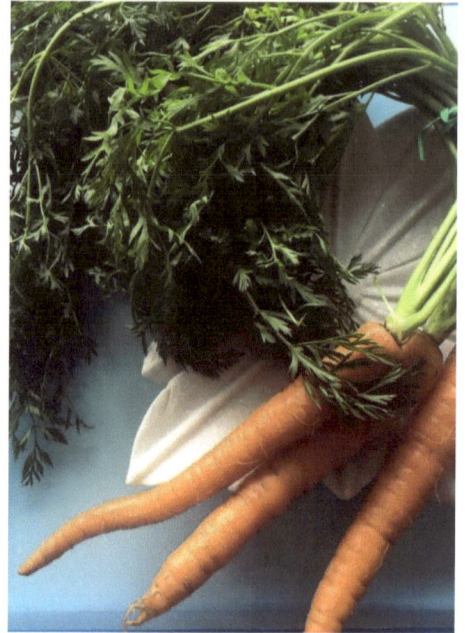

Health Benefits of Carrots

1. Carotenoids in carrots reduce the risk of heart disease.

2. Eating six or more carrots a week will reduce the possibility of a stroke.

3. Carbohydrates in the carrots reduce the amount of the body's cholesterol.

4. Carotenoids found in carrots have anti-cancer effects.

5. Smokers who do not consume carrots are more likely to have lung cancer than those who eat carrots more than once a week.

6. Studies in Japan have shown that beta-carotenoids in carrots reduce the likelihood of colon cancer.

7. Carrot juice kills leukemia cells and inhibits their progression.

8. Carbohydrates in carrots facilitate digestive processes and maintain intestinal cleansing.

9. If you have a cold or sore throat, try gargling with a mixture of 0.4 tablespoon of warm boiled carrot juice and 1 tablespoon of honey.

10. In case of stomatitis, it is advisable to rinse your mouth with fresh carrot juice.

11. If you suffer from constipation, drink 150 to 200 ml of fresh carrot juice before eating, or grate one carrot, add a teaspoon of olive oil, and mix. Eat purée before bedtime.

12. The antioxidants in carrots can help slow down the aging processes, strengthen the immune system, and regulate the amount of sugar.

13. Carrot juice is recommended for those having heart, kidney, or liver problems. They revitalize and soften the skin. Their masks are excellent for maintaining healthy facial skin. It is recommended to drink the juice immediately, and if you do not manage to drink the juice in one go, put it in a glass container and keep it in the refrigerator for no more than 2-3 hours.

14. If you eat unpeeled carrots, the body absorbs only 5% of carotene on average, whereas it absorbs over four times more from grated carrots.

15. In folk medicine, frostbites, wounds, and ulcers are treated with grated carrot compresses.

16. A face mask made from carrot helps to refresh and soften the skin. To do this, grate one carrot mixed with 1 teaspoon of honey, 1 teaspoon of olive oil, and a few teaspoons of lemon juice. Rub the face with this mixture and gently massage. Leave the face mask for 5 minutes and then rinse with warm water. Do not forget that carrots dye the skin, so it is better to enjoy their masks for no more than 5 minutes. Before putting the mask on the face, consider your skin type.

Carrot Balls

Ingredients:
- 10 carrots,
- 3 apples,
- ½ glass of semolina,
- 1 egg,
- ½ glass of breadcrumbs or flour,
- sugar,
- salt,
- 1 tablespoon of butter,
- ½ glass of milk.

Preparation: Grate the washed and peeled carrots and apples (put into a beetroot grater). Next, put them in a pot, add a little water, milk, butter, and cook until it gets smooth, then add semolina, sugar, salt, and egg. Mix well, shape the mixture into balls, cover them with breadcrumbs, and bake in well-heated butter.

Before serving, sprinkle them with butter or sour cream, or butter and sour cream sauce.

Pancakes Made from Farmer Cheese and Flour with Carrots

Ingredients:
- 4 carrots,
- 500kg (1 pound) of curd,
- 1 egg,
- 1 tablespoon of butter,
- 2 tablespoons of semolina,
- ½ cup of flour, salt,
- 1 tablespoon of sugar.

Preparation: Slice and wash the carrots, cut them into cubes and stew with a small amount of water and butter.

Grind the stewed carrots in a meat grinder or mash through a sieve, add semolina, curd, egg, salt, sugar, and flour.

After mixing, make round breads and fry in a frying pan with butter, first on one side and then on the other.

Serve with sour cream.

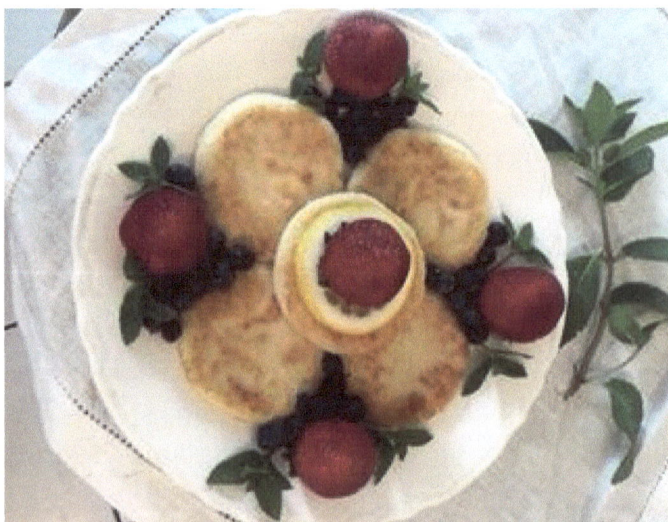

Those "Unnecessary" Carrot Leaves…

1. The use of carrot leaves is unusual for us. We always throw them away without thinking about their significant benefits. They are also very rich in vitamins and minerals.
2. Carrot leaves are no less useful than root beet leaves. They can be put in soups, salads, marinated as vegetables, and even drunk as a tea. Ladies who drink tea from dried carrot leaves throughout the winter will be amazed at the look of their legs. Their hated blue-veins disappear to their joy and amazement. Carrot leaf juice helps to treat thrombophlebitis and hemorrhoids.
3. Our grandmothers used carrot leaf rinse on their hair. It greatly enhances and strengthens the hair and stimulates their growth.
4. A compressed decoction from carrot leaves helps psoriasis, dermatitis, and allergic rash.
5. The property of carrot leaves is to tone up and help them get rid of blood clots.

Add carrot leaf to your food: Wash the carrot leaves and chop them like parsley. Next, dry them and add to your salads or casseroles. They will not affect the taste until cooked, but the benefits will be huge.

Dried **carrot leaf tea** is useful and can improve vision, cleanse the blood, and treat colds. Put a handful of dried leaves in a teapot, pour boiling water into it, and leave it to stand in a covered teapot for about 30 minutes. It is advisable to drink without any additives.

Carrot leaves are harvested in June and July when they have the most beneficial microelements. After harvesting, wash, drain, finely chop, and put them on clean shade or white paper for drying in a well-ventilated room. When the leaflets are completely dry, put them in jars and close them with tight caps. They will be suitable for use for about one year, preserving all medicinal properties.

Cucumber

Cucumber (Cucumis sativus) originates from India where it was first grown at least 3000 years ago. The Ancient Egyptians ate them with each meal. Caravans traveling through the deserts would carry cucumbers to quench their thirst. During the summer heats, the Greeks cooled themselves by lying on finely-cut cucumbers. The Roman Empire could not stand without cucumber for at least one day; they ate them green, boiled, and with oil, honey, or vinegar. According to one story, the Emperor Tiberius ate 10 cucumbers every day. In England, cucumbers were popularized by Henry VIII. They were used in folk medicine to cure the flu. The doctor would instruct the patient to lay down on cut cucumbers. Dog bites were also treated with cucumber leaves filled with wine.

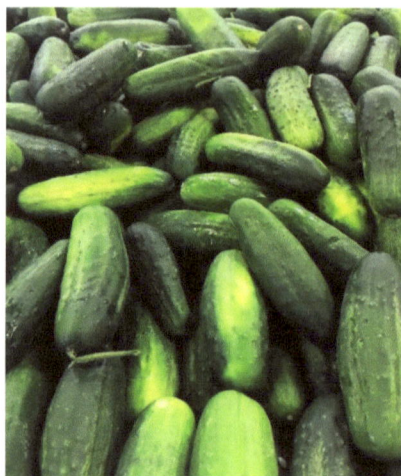

Cucumbers are a refreshing summer vegetable, comprised of 95% water. The gourd contains proteins, sugar, (fructose and glucose), vitamins C, E, B1, B2, B6, PP, A, minerals, and iodine. These vitamins and minerals help to improve the thyroid function, memory, and strengthen blood vessels. Early cucumbers have a lot of vitamin C and it is a low-calorie fruit. Cucumbers have special enzymes that help to absorb animal proteins. Therefore, nutritionists recommend eating meat and fish products with salad containing cucumbers.

Cucumber Health Benefits

1. Cucumbers dissolve stones, destroy microbes, strengthen the heart, and help to eliminate toxins.
2. It is recommended to eat cucumbers when you suffer from diabetes, atherosclerosis, kidney, liver, heart, and small intestine diseases, as well as being overweight or having constipation.
3. In summer, try to eat more cucumbers. You will find that your face color will improve, your nails will strengthen, and more glossy hair will grow.
4. The silicon and sulfur present in cucumbers will improve the condition of the teeth and gums.
5. In cosmetics, cucumbers are used to smooth wrinkles and to close the skin pores. The juice soothes and moisturizes dry, shiny skin. Cleansing the skin with cucumber juice makes the skin softer, whiter, and freckles and pigmentation spots disappear.

Cucumber applications: Thinly slice a cucumber and grease your face with its juice. It is best to do this in the evening before going to bed. If your facial or body skin has acne, drink a glass of cucumber juice every day. If you put the cuttings of the cucumber on your face and under your eyes, you will eliminate fine lines.

Eat one cucumber each day or eat 1.5 kg of fresh cucumbers per day on your "Cucumber Day". You can drink ½ a liter of fresh buttermilk with cucumbers.

If your skin is dry, grease with grated cucumber puree, keep it for about half an hour, and wipe it with a cotton swab

Cucumbers grow well in large pots; you will need to support them or sow bush cucumbers.

Cucumbers need to be harvested during the full moon, as this is when they are most delicious.

Freshly picked cucumbers eaten with honey are very refreshing in the summer.

People who have allergies to seeds, honey, or spices **should not use cucumbers.** You can replace these ingredients with other ingredients

Fresh Summer Salad

Ingredients: 3 green cucumbers, 1 carrot, 1 cooked beetroot, 1 tablespoon of sesame seeds, 1 tablespoon of sunflower seeds, ½ lemon juice, 1 slice of pineapple, 2 cloves of garlic, 3 tablespoons of olive oil, spices of your choice.

Preparation: Grate cucumbers, carrot, cooked beetroot, slice pineapple, add sunflower, sesame seeds, crushed garlic, and other additives. Mix everything well.

Pickled Cucumbers in the Bag

Ingredients:
- 500 g of cucumbers,
- three cloves of garlic,
- 1 handful of diced dills,
- 1 teaspoon of salt.

Preparation: cut freshly picked cucumbers into four parts, chop finely the garlic and dill. Put everything in a cellophane bag with a zipper, put a teaspoon of salt and shake well. Put in the refrigerator. Eat after half an hour.

.

Chapter 6

TREES

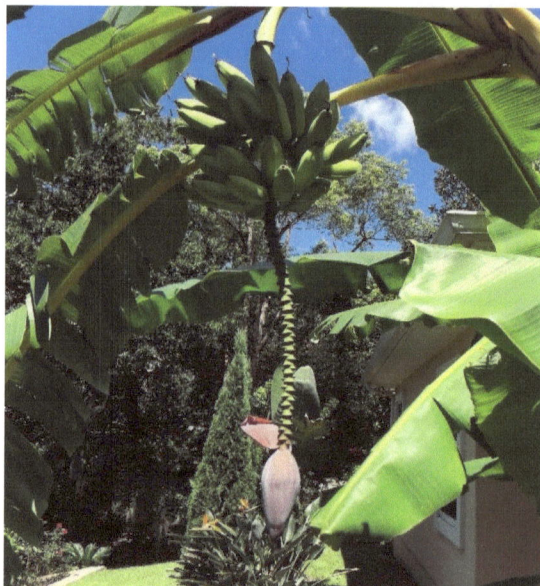

Close to the gates a spacious garden lies,
From the storms and inclement skies;
Four acres was the allotted space of ground,
Fenc'd with a green enclosure all around.
Tall thriving tree confessed the fruitful mold:
The reddening apple ripens here to gold,
Here the blue fig with luscious juice overflows,
With deeper red the full pomegranate glows,
The branch here bends beneath the weighty pear,
and verdant olives flourish round the year.
Homer, Odyssey, circa 850 B. C.

Trees not only decorate the environment, but they also cleanse the air from dust, absorb harmful substances, and emit decontaminated air into the environment. Their emitted volatile substances combine with contaminant molecules and excrete themselves from the environment. Thus, we are not only provided with fresh air but also with ionized air due to the trees.

Smells diffused by plants regulate microflora and effect our immune system. The easiest way to take advantage of these natural opportunities is to take a walk in a forest or park and to breathe their healing aromas. The trees protect from soil erosion. They carry out photosynthesis and create a large amount of substances and regulate airflow by absorbing giant amount of carbon dioxide. Scientists claim that trees help to recover lost strengths as they emit a strong bioenergy. Such trees are easy to distinguish because other trees cannot grow as tall as them, with heights of 5-6 meters (1 meter is equal to 39 inches) and become stunted when planted or sprouted because of the energy of a strong neighbor.

The full moon, the new moon, and the eclipses are not the proper time to use tree energy. A waning moon is suitable for removing energies, and a waxing moon is suitable for loading them. Different trees affect people in different ways with their abilities to calm, heal, supplement energy, and remove stress.

The oak tree has a high bioenergetic power. When a person receives the maximum amount of vital energy during direct contact with this tree, it strengthens immunity, heals infectious diseases, improves mood, activates brain activity, provides strength, enlivens blood circulation, and helps people to recover faster. This is a tree of art and prophecy—it is a symbol of longevity, power, and strength across the whole of Europe. Even people with severe illnesses should interact with this tree.

The oak is the tree of fighters. It can not only strengthen but also load vital energy, and even change the mindset. Parapsychologists say that you must go with good thoughts if you want to get energy from the oak tree. When you feel a positive energy from the oak, stand for 5 to 6 minutes pressing against the bark with your back, because the energy is absorbed through the spinal cord.

Tree fruits have a lot of biologically-active substances that can protect against chronic tumors, malignant tumors, and cardiovascular diseases, etc. The adult person should eat about 300g of fruit per day. The best time to eat fruit is half an hour before a meal and to start the day with a glass of water. Then, eat an apple with half a glass of berries. If you eat 2 apples a day, it will fulfill your needed daily fruit intake.

You need to follow your intuition when you are eating fruit. You may have noticed that when you start eating it is very delicious, and then the taste starts to change; this is a sign that you do not need to eat it anymore.

People who are allergic to fruit should not overuse them.

Dates

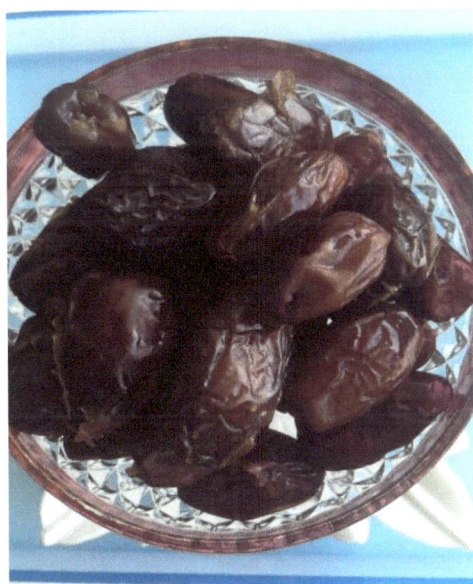

Date palm (Phoenix dactylifera). Dates are also called the desert bread. It is known that dates have been used by the Arabs as far back as seven thousand years ago. Dried fruits rich in minerals and various sugars are one of the main Bedouin food products; so it goes without saying as to why the Arabs refer to date palms as dessert bread. Archaeologists have established that the palms of dates were traditionally grown in Ancient Egypt, Assyria, Babylon, and in Sumerian settlements because this palm can grow in wintry desert conditions into long-lasting nutritious fruits. Date trees were called "blessed trees," and later became the ancient Jewish emblem. Date palms symbolized fertility and God's generosity. Since ancient times, one of the greatest sins was to cut the palm of a matured fruit. The average height of a date palm tree is 25 meters, and about

80 kg of fruit are usually collected from such trees every year. Botanists have found a total of 15 breeds of date palm trees, and there are many more kinds and subspecies. The dates, depending on the kind, can range in color from white to black.

Beer, garlic, and a handful of dates was the daily intake of the pyramid builders. The beer satisfied the body's fluid needs, the garlic overcame infections, and the dried date fruit provided the energy needed to work such hard and exhausting physical work.

This ancient candy is useful for children and adults. Dates are rich in iron, phosphorus, mineral salts, and vitamins. Ten dates are enough to meet the daily needs of magnesium, copper, and sulfur in the human body. The same ten dates comprise half the amount of the daily human body needs for calcium and iron.

Health Benefits of Dates

Physicians recommend dates for pregnant women, since the dates contain substances that strengthen the muscles of the uterus in the last months of pregnancy. Dates not only facilitate birth, but they also help to recover from it more quickly. In addition, the dates enrich the breast milk with the most important vitamins. However, due to constipation, the pregnant women should consume fewer than 8 dates a day.

The Arabs always regarded dates as drugs. Dates contain almost all of the body's required vitamins, except E and H. In particular, they accumulate plenty of vitamin B5, thus improving the capacity for work and increasing concentration.

The substances found in dates are very similar to aspirin in structure. For this reason, the oracles probably used them for healing colds and relieving headaches.

The Arab popular phrase "Eat the dates, save your tooth," has been justified with scientific research because they contain substances that protect your teeth from caries.

Dates do not have cholesterol and have low calories. One fruit contains only about 23 calories, and it takes only a few dates to satisfy an appetite.

With plenty of magnesium, dates can help a number of very serious illnesses, such as intestine cancer. They also help in healing paralysis and protecting sight and hearing.

Dates are recommended to eat if you have nervous system disorders or heart, blood vessel, or respiratory tract diseases. Dried date fruits are irreplaceable for physically exhausted organisms. They return strength, strengthen the bones, and stimulate muscle functioning.

It is necessary not to forget that dates take a long time to digest, therefore, dates are **not recommended** to eat for those with gastrointestinal tract disorders. They also contain a lot of carbohydrates, so people who are overweight or with diabetes should avoid them.

Pomegranates

Pomegranates (Punica granatum) are also called royal fruits. In Babylon, pomegranates began growing about 5000 BC. Pomegranates are probably the oldest cultivated fruit tree. In India, pomegranate juice is called "the health elixir," while the ancient Egyptians regarded pomegranates as a symbol of love, fertility, and well-being. According to Greek legend Aphrodite, the goddess of love and beauty, planted pomegranates on the island of Cyprus. From then on, pomegranates symbolized love and fertility for these nations.

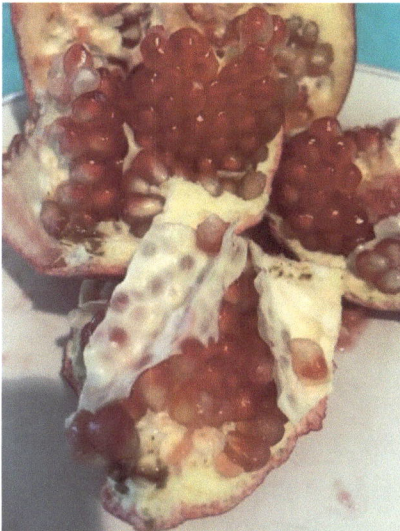

One of the oldest medical records indicates that Egyptians used pomegranates to treat tapeworm infections. The ancient Greek physician Hippocrates (460-377) advised drinking pomegranate juice while treating gastric pains and to use the peel to prevent long-lasting diarrhea and to treat dysentery or internal wounds. Tibetan physicians treated gastrointestinal tract diseases, kidney colic pains, and diabetes with pomegranate juice. They also used it to heal scurvy and burns with evaporated juice. In addition, they strengthened their body and quenched their thirst with this juice.

Ayurveda recommends pomegranates to satisfy thirst during a fever. Pomegranate seeds and juice are regarded as a tonic of the heart and a dissolver of cholesterol in arteries. In 2004, scientists declared that a glass of pomegranate juice a day can completely stop atherosclerosis and even treat it.

Health Benefits of Pomegranates

Pomegranates improve intelligence and memory and help to maintain a mental and physical balance.

Ayurveda claims that pomegranates remove impotence. The man should eat one fruit every evening for 14 days. Pomegranate and ginger juice mixed with honey will help to cure coughs and bronchitis. Drink 4-5 teaspoons every 3 hours.

Pomegranate juice is a great natural ayurvedic remedy for gastric ulcers.

Pomegranate juice has an antibacterial effect. Viral infections can be suppressed with pomegranate juice and its extracts.

Fresh pomegranate juice is a great antioxidant that protects against free radicals, inhibits the aging process, suppresses the development of cancer cells, and enhances immunity in the treatment of AIDS. Pomegranates also stop the formation of unnecessary blood clots, and it is believed that pomegranates slow the development of cataracts.

Scientific research shows that pomegranate extracts can protect against osteoarthritis. The pomegranate is rich in vitamin C and potassium, and it is a good source of low-calorie intake.

The inside of the pomegranate contains between 200 and 1200 seeds covered by a red juicy layer. This layer can be eaten and is used in cooking, for it is rich in minerals and vitamins. The vitamin B6 contained in the pomegranate protects the muscles from cramps and pain caused by physical exertions. In addition, this vitamin helps to absorb magnesium.

If you spend a lot of time on your computer, vitamin PP contained in the pomegranate protects the sight, which is very helpful in an increasingly digital world. This vitamin also reduces the cholesterol levels in the blood. Pomegranate seeds are rich in iron, therefore, it is useful to eat fresh fruit and drink juice in order to increase the amount of hemoglobin in the blood.

Pomegranates contain fiber, natural sugar, carbohydrates, proteins, iron, calcium, vitamin C, zinc, potassium, phosphorus, magnesium, and the following group B vitamins: B1 (thiamine), B2 (niacin), B3 (riboflavin), B9 (folic acid), B5, B6 (pantothenic acid).

Daily intake of pomegranate juice is very useful for people suffering from low blood pressure and asthma. Pomegranate juice also cleans the blood. Drink 200 ml every day in the evening and before sleeping. The juice reduces fever, inflammation of the gastrointestinal tract in the stomach and intestines, and removes bad odor in the mouth. Pomegranate juices are very helpful in relieving diarrhea, but excessive amounts can cause constipation.

Pomegranate juices are good for women to control the risk of breast cancer. This is a preventive measure against Alzheimer's disease, and juice is suitable for treatment as it slows the process of the disease.

Pomegranates should be avoided. Although allergies caused by pomegranate are very rare, in some people it appears as skin irritation and burning sensation, so they should avoid this fruit. The acidity of the pomegranate fruit may aggravate symptoms of heartburn; in this case, do not eat or drink the pomegranate juice before going to sleep. You also need to limit vitamin K consumption if you have thin blood because this vitamin suppresses blood clotting.

When drinking pomegranate juice, it is necessary to dilute with water because it contains a variety of acids that burn the stomach and remove the tooth enamel.

Pomegranates in Cosmetics

Pomegranate peels are widely used in cosmetics to treat the face and scalp for seborrhea and burns. It is advisable to rinse your hair with a cleanser of fruit peels to make the hair grow faster.

Acid contained in the pomegranate removes pigmented spots, freckles, and acne.
Sweet fruit juice mixed with sour cream in equal parts perfectly whitens and nourishes dry and normal facial skin.

Persimmons

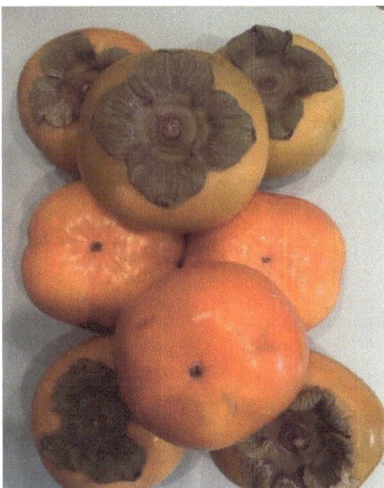

Persimmon (diospyros). If you translate the word persimmon in Greek, "dios" and "pyron", you get "Food of the Gods." Persimmon is also called churma, which translated from Turkish means "sweet sweet."

The homeland of the persimmon is China, and from there it spread throughout East Asia, and then later into Japan. By the end of the 19th century these fruits had spread all over the world. Eastern countries call the persimmon the orange sun, the Philippines call persimmon "mabolo," and in Italy it is called "kaki." The name persimmon came from the Red Indian languages where it was called "puchtamine," "pasiminan," "pesmine," and "persimmon."

It is said that persimmons can withstand even 27°C to 30°C degrees of cold. The tree lives 100-150 years, grows 5-10 meters high, and enjoys deep roots. The fruit is ripe during the September-November months. They give a good crop every year and the fruits are usually harvested unripe.

Persimmons contain high levels of vitamin A, C, P, carotene, and many microelements such as potassium, magnesium, iron, iodine, copper, and calcium. Persimmons do not have many calories—100g of persimmon contains only 60 kcal.

Health Benefits of Persimmons

Persimmons have a diuretic effect and help to lessen coughs. The carotene contained in persimmons protects the eyesight and slows down the pace of aging. Persimmons are suitable for those who suffer from digestive disorders or diarrhea. The persimmon is valued in the diet of elderly people because it reduces arterial blood pressure, strengthens the bloodstream, and helps the body to recover from physical exhaustion.

High levels of sugar (almost 18%) consisting of glucose and fructose support the cardiovascular system and feed the heart muscle, but glucose levels do not increase dangerously in the blood.

Persimmons calm the nervous system, increase work capacity, and reduce headaches. Persimmons are useful for losing weight and to control your appetite—a high amount of fiber helps to get rid of hunger for a long time.

You should pay attention to a few of these nuances when eating:

Diabetics should not eat lots of persimmons because they have high levels of sugar. People with anemia should be aware that high levels of tannin can inhibit iron absorption. Those who suffer from gastritis should avoid eating persimmons because of those same tannin acids. It is better to avoid eating persimmons during constipation. Persimmons should be eaten after a meal. If you eat them on an empty stomach, stones can be formed in the body. Do not eat more than 3 persimmons at one time. Clean teeth and rinse the throat after eating persimmons because the acids can damage your teeth. Nutritionists advise peeling a persimmon before eating.

If you tend to have allergies, be careful with persimmon, as it is a very allergic fruit.

Persimmon salad with Apples and Pomegranates.

Ingredients: 1 persimmon, 1 apple, pomegranate seeds, a few mint leaves, ½ teaspoon of lemon juice, a tablespoon of honey.

Preparation: Cut the persimmon and apple into cubes. Mix everything thoroughly, pour the pomegranate seeds on the top, decorate with mint leaves, and pour honey mixed with lemon juice.

Banana

Banana (Musa). The banana was one of the first fruits planted by the human being in India. Cultivated 3500 years ago, the banana is a highly fragrant fruit that is rich in minerals and fiber.

Banana peel is a great fertilizer. To make the roses grow well and flower, place banana peels down before planting.

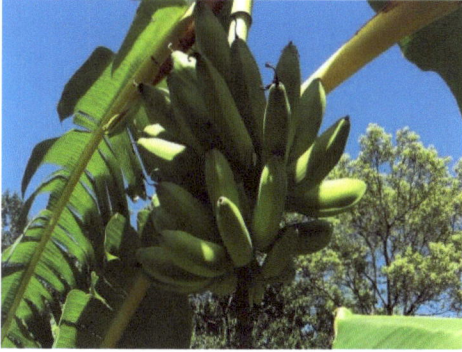

The banana is the fosterer of youth and the enemy of aging.

You can get your daily requirement of potassium by eating two bananas. It's best to eat them in small quantities on a regular basis to achieve the best results.

Nutritionists advise eating bananas both before and after training, allowing the body to quickly absorb the necessary energy.

Health Benefits of Bananas

Bananas contain a lot of vitamins, minerals, and fiber. They are rich in iron, thus useful for treating anemia. Iron is used in the production of hemoglobin in our red cells. Bananas reduce kidney stone formation. They reduce stomach acidity and help with gastritis, ulcers, and heartburn symptoms, and a variety of other digestive tract disorders.

Reduce insect bite irritation by greasing them with the inner side of the banana peel.

The pectin in bananas eases constipation.

Group B vitamins in bananas help to soothe the nervous system, improve concentration, combat stress, protect against depression, and activate mental activity.

Bananas have a positive effect on the kidneys and improve the skin's condition. The banana is a good food for babies because it does not cause allergies.

Bananas are **not recommended** for people on diets because they are quite caloric. Bananas are also not recommended for people with diabetes because they contain sucrose, which stimulates the secretion of sugar in the blood.

Banana Pancakes

These pancakes are naturally sweet because there is no flour or gluten in them, and they do not contain fat or added sugar. Many consider these pancakes to be the healthiest in the world. In addition, these pancakes are easy to make.

Ingredients:
1 ripe banana,
2 eggs,
¼ teaspoon of baking soda.
If you want, add chopped nuts, raisins, or cinnamon to the dough.
Preparation: Blend the banana until the mass is homogeneous without small lumps. Put eggs in the banana mass, add the baking soda, and mix well. Bake in a frying pan until they get crispy. These pancakes are stacked on top of each other by serving banana crumbs on the top. Eat with yogurt, maple syrup, or honey.

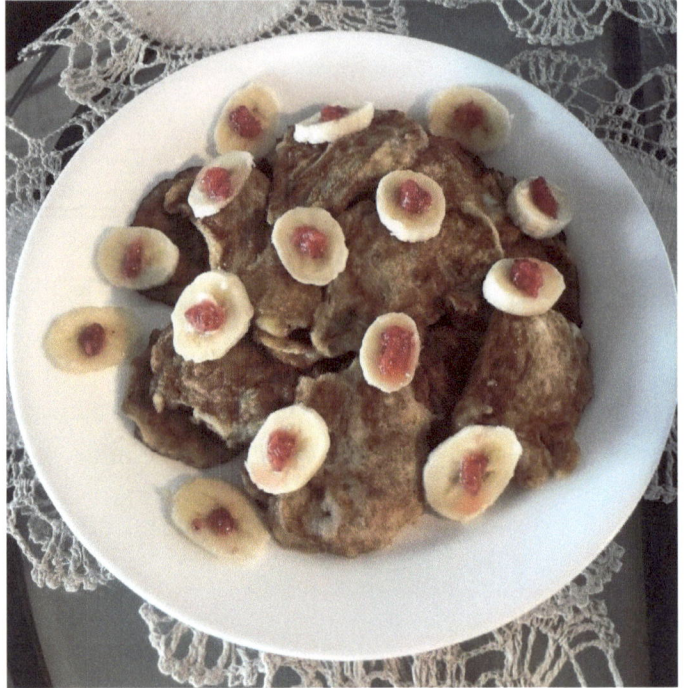

Honey, nuts, and cinnamon may bother those with allergies.

Avocado

Avocado (Persea americana). Avocado is a fruit mainly grown in South America on deciduous trees of 20 meters height. Originating in Central America, it is one of the most valued fruits in the world with many beneficial nutrients. The avocado is rich in vitamins (11 types), minerals (14 types), proteins, carbohydrates, and up to 32% fat. It is best known as the main ingredient in preparing Mexican guacamole.

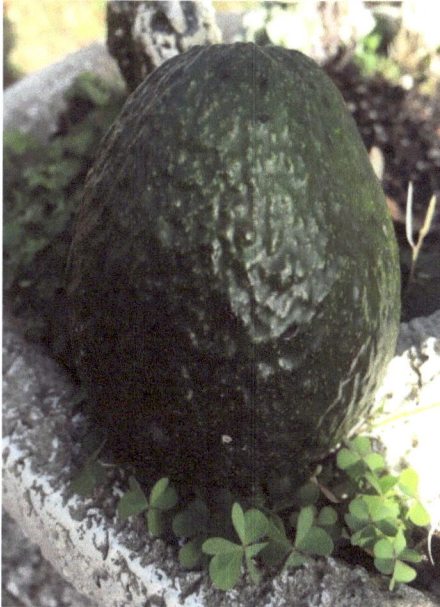

The fruit comes in the form of a green pear with a large stone between 7-20 cm in length, weighing from 250 g to 600 g.

The avocado is eaten when it is completely ripe and a pitfall appears in the hole. If the fruit is hard, keep for one day or a few days at room temperature and it will ripe.

The fastest way to ripen an avocado is to place it in a paper bag with a banana or an apple. Those fruits secrete ethylene which aids the avocado maturation. In this way, avocados ripen in about a day.

Eat a prepared fruit as soon as possible because it dries out easily losing a lot of its useful substances. The most valuable fruits are dark green in color and have rough skins. They contain a lot of vitamins and minerals.

Avocado is suitable for salads, cold snacks, or sauces. The fruit is quickly digested.

Health Benefits of Avocado

Avocado is rich in dietary fiber. If you eat a medium-sized avocado, you get almost half of the daily recommended dietary fiber. Avocado is also rich in vegetable proteins and has a low amount of sugar. In addition to its caloric content, avocado is great for those who stay on diet. Avocado stimulates the regeneration of the skin and hair, fights small wrinkles, and is ideal for facial masks.

Avocado is suitable for prophylaxis of heart and blood vessel diseases, and furthermore:

- It has a positive effect on the brain and nervous system.
- It improves metabolism.

- It protects the liver from accumulation of fat by dissolving excess fat in the body.
- Avocado reduces the amount of sugar in the blood.
- It helps to protect from cancer.
- Avocado improves vascular elasticity.
- Avocado is important for people who suffer from high levels of cholesterol in the blood.

How to Make Guacamole

Guacamole is a sauce of Mexican origin. The main ingredient is avocado. This is an excellent sauce with a mild taste, and is especially suitable for eating with corn chips.

Ingredients:
2 ripe avocados,
½ teaspoon of mineral (Himalayan) salt,
1 teaspoon of lemon or lime juice,
2-4 tablespoons of crushed red onion (to taste),
1-2 chopped Serrano chili pepper (small, spicy, multicolored, bullet-shaped pepper) without seeds and stems,
2 tablespoons of chopped coriander,
black pepper to taste,
half of one ripe sunburned tomato without peel.

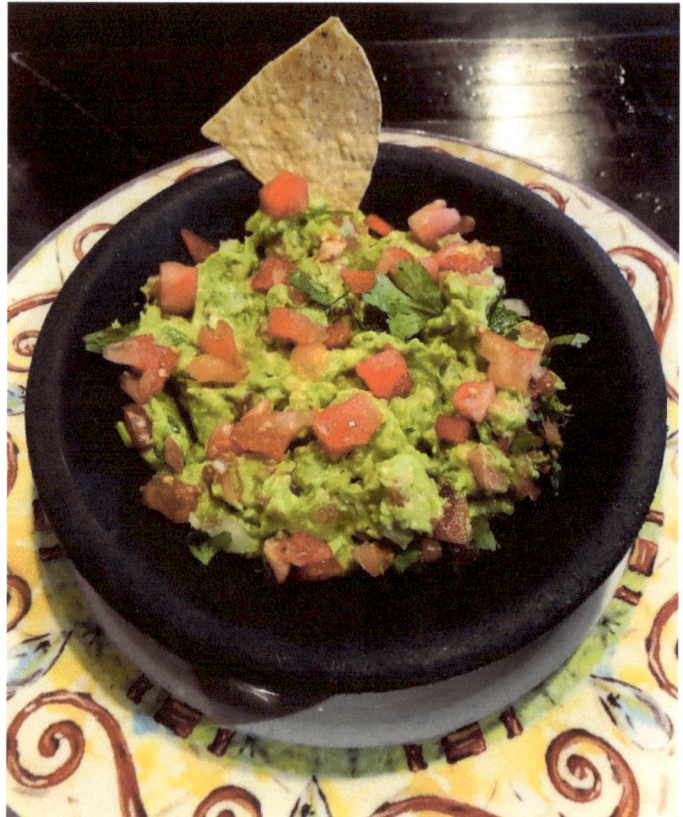

Preparation: Peel the avocado and remove the stone. Crush the fruit in a bowl and add the remaining ingredients, mixing well. It's important to be cautious with the chili peppers – some are hotter than others!

Apple

Apple (Pome). This is one of the most popular and healthiest of the fruits. It prolongs life and protects against various illnesses.

"An apple a day keeps the doctor away." – English Folk saying

Apples contain a lot of fiber, which lowers blood cholesterol levels, helps to improve digestion, and inhibits the development of diabetes mellitus. Vitamin C is rich in apples; it protects children from various infections, helps the body to absorb iron, stimulates collagen production, and acts as an antioxidant. The apple contains Group B vitamins that revitalize the skin. Pectins present in the apple help to eliminate toxins and avoid constipation. A glass of apple juice a day is an excellent preventive measure for heart disease. One medium-sized apple has 80 calories.

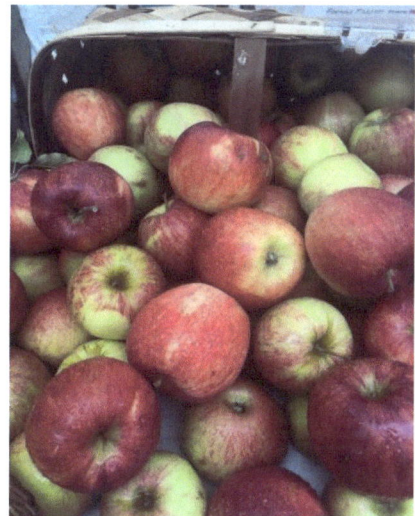

Health Benefits of Apples

Research shows that eating an apple every day reduces the amount of bad cholesterol in the blood because they contain pectin, actually keeping the doctor (cardiologist) away.

Apples help to digest other foods.
Apples protect bones.
Apples strengthen the immune system.
Health experts say that apples can protect from a variety of cancer types; including breast, lung, liver, pancreas, and colon.
Eating two apples a day, you will make it easier to lose weight.
To keep your teeth healthy and beautiful, eat apples.
Apples protect from bladder stones.
The apple peel has plenty of useful substances for the body, so do not peel the apple.

Cellulite. Cut two apples halfway and add to boiling water. When they cool down, massage the problematic areas with the apple halves. Next, wash your skin with water and apply moisturizing cream. Even after the first procedure, the skin will become more elastic. The thighs can be thinner by up to 2 cm in one month. Do not forget that the results will only depend on you. Regular exercise for the legs and buttocks will help to get rid of cellulite even faster.

Recipes:

Oatmeal Flakes with Grated Apples
The loveliest breakfast in winter, it is a perfect meal for adults—delicious and nutritious, and with lots of fiber.
Ingredients:
1 cup of oatmeal,
2½ cups of water,
a pinch of salt,
1 medium size apple grated in large cubes,
½ tbsp lemon juice,
½ cup of milk,
½ teaspoon of butter.
Preparation: Mix the oatmeal, water, and salt in a small saucepan. Boil and add the grated apple. Cook until the porridge thickens. Add the butter, milk and lemon juice, and mix thoroughly. Serve hot and sprinkle with brown sugar or maple syrup.

Baked Apples
Ingredients:
¼ cup of crushed walnuts,
4 apples (Cortland, Golden Delicious, or Rome Beauty),
4 teaspoons of butter,
4 teaspoons of sugar
½ teaspoon of cinnamon,
2 tablespoons of water.
Preparation: Wash the apples and remove the core. Place them on a greased baking dish.
Mix butter, sugar, cinnamon, and crushed walnuts and pour into the center of the apples. Add water to the pan.
Bake the apples for 30 minutes in a preheated oven at 350 F, (180°C). Serve warm.
Additional serving suggestions: Add a dollop of yogurt just before serving, and/or pour some maple syrup or honey on top and decorate with a mint twig or blossom of a flower.

Citrus Fruits

All citrus fruits come from the Rutaceae family. During the renaissance, oranges protected people from the plague, and this fruit was considered an herb. Ludwig XIV cultivated oranges in a glass hothouse in Versailles Park. In the palace, ladies would take orange decoction baths because it gave shyness to the skin. Doctors also recommended rubbing teeth and gums with citrus fruits. Citrus fruits have always been used to enhance health and improve beauty even when their benefits to the body had not yet been scientifically validated.

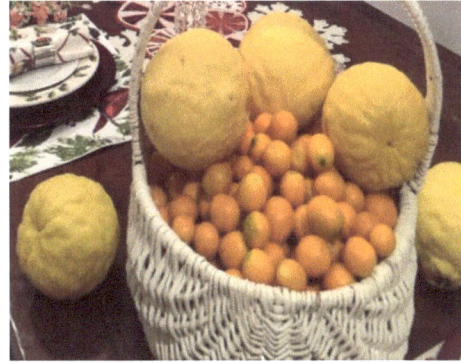

Health Benefits of Citrus Fruits

Orange (Citrus:sinensis). Oranges improve appetite and digestion, reduce the risk of cancer, and regulate blood sugar. The essential oils in orange peel give it a pleasant smell.

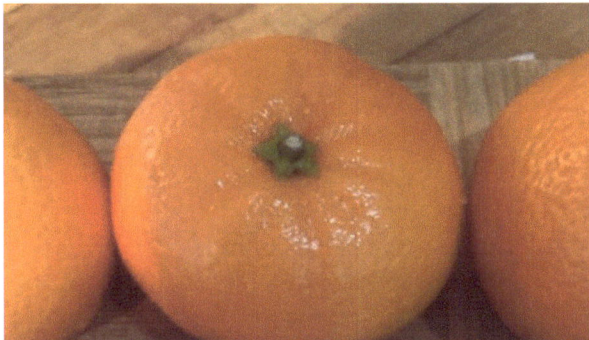

Orange juice is a great source of vitamin C, especially during the warm seasons. Juice strengthens immunity, provides strength and energy, improves the development of the body, removal of waste, and cleaves fats well, thus helping to combat obesity. Oranges promote the removal of excess salts accumulated in the body.

Grapefruit (Citrus:paradisi). The film covering each lobe is a source of bioflavonoids that strengthens the blood vessels and helps to absorb vitamin C. The grapefruit improves appetite and digestion and is an excellent remedy against stress and low moods.

Grapefruit juice is a great source of vitamin C, increases the body's resistance to diseases, helps to overcome fatigue, and lowers arterial pressure. Grapefruit juice reduces cholesterol in the blood and dissolves salts.

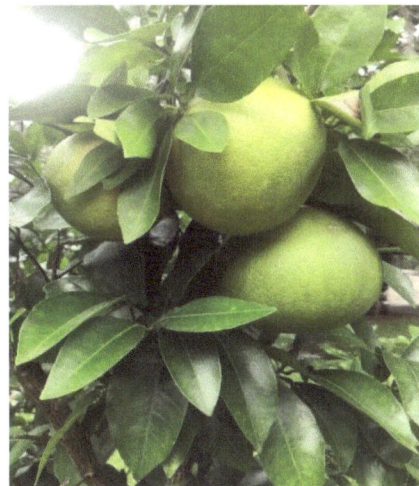

Mandarin (Citrus:reticulata). Mandarins not only contain vitamin C but also vitamin D, which reduces the risk of rickets. Mandarins also improve vascular elasticity and are recommended to eat for those suffering from stomach disease and intestinal disorders.

Lemon

Lemon (Citrus:limon). It is believed that lemons originated from the Himalayan Mountains located in the east of India and then spread around the world, growing best in temperate and tropical climates. The lime (or green lemon) is smaller than the lemon and less sour. The lemon is one of the most widely used fruits in the world.

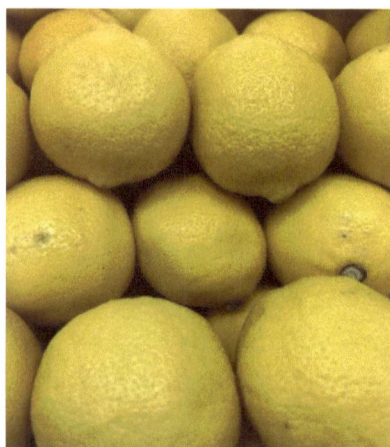

Sailors and researchers began using lemons in the 18th century, when they had to spend a long time on board without fresh fruits or vegetables. At that time, sailors often suffered from scurvy (vitamin C deficiency), sight disorders, gum bleeding, and teeth falling out. In 1747, Scott James Lind established that lemons and oranges could help avoid scurvy and treat it. By the end of the 18th century, the English navy had declared that every sailor had to drink 30ml of lemon juice daily. Nowadays, lemons are used for flavoring teas, salad dressings, garnishes, marinades, desserts, and drinks.

Health Benefits of Lemons

Vitamin C, a powerful antioxidant found in lemon juice, neutralizes free radicals and protects against cancer. Lemons have antimicrobial effects against bacteria and fungal infections. They are also effective against parasites and worms, and regulate blood pressure if it is too high. The lemon is an antidepressant and helps those struggling with stress and nervous disorders.

Vitamin C is extremely important for maintaining the immune system, producing white blood cells, and delaying premature aging. Vitamin C plays an important role in collagen production, which is responsible for skin elasticity and improving skin structure. Eating foods that contain high levels of vitamin C and iron will maximize iron absorption to prevent and treat anemia.

Lemon Use for Beauty

Rinse hair with lemon juice to have shiny hair.

Dry and weak nails will be strengthened by mixing lemon juice with olive oil, and nourishing nails in it. Lemon juice is applied to scars from old burns, juice can help reduce or eliminate them. Juice also whitens the skin.

Amazing Frozen Lemons

Lemon peel contains 5-10 times more vitamins than lemon juice. We tend to throw the peel without thinking, but lemon peel is a strong toxicity-reducing agent.

Wash and dry your older lemon and put it in the freezer. When the lemon is frozen, grate the whole lemon with the peel. All the products you make will have a fresh taste with added lemon peel. Sprinkle the grated lemons on salad, ice, soups, porridges, macaroni, spaghetti, rice, sushi, and fish dishes. They even can spice up whiskey and wine.

Lemon, Ginger, and Mint Drink
Ingredients:
2 liters of drinking water (2000) ml,
1 slice of lemon, mint leaves to taste,
1 teaspoon of minced ginger,
1 cucumber without peel cut into slices.
Preparation: Mix everything in the jug and put it in a refrigerator. It will be a refreshing summer drink in the morning.

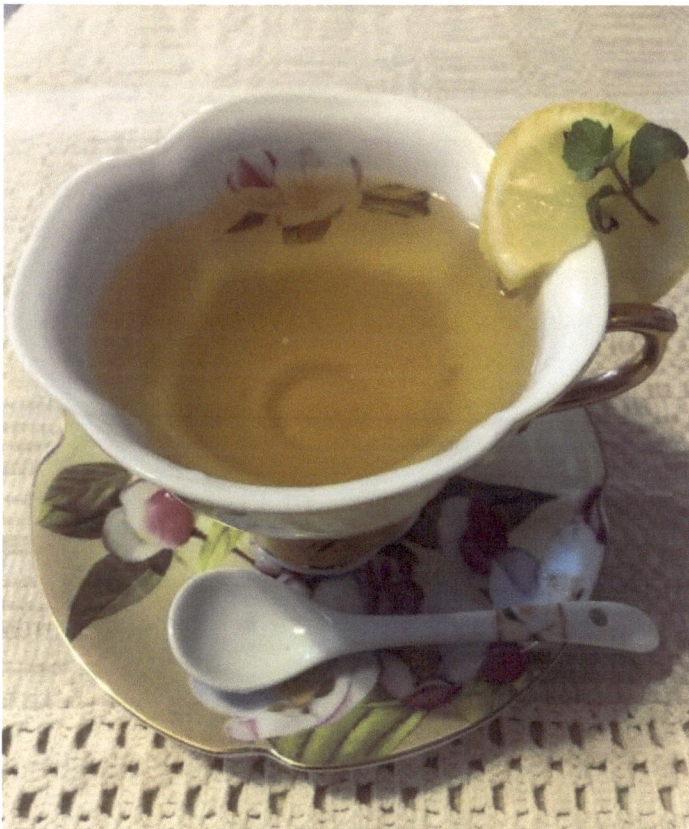

Lemon and Honey Drink
Ingredients:
A glass of warm but not boiling water,
½ lemon juice,
1 teaspoon of honey.
Preparation: Boil the water, cool a bit, put all ingredients together, stir and drink in the morning before the meal. (You can add a slice of ginger to the boiling water).

Chapter 17

NUTS

Small brown, hard, round,
The nut is lying underground.
Now a shoot begins to show.
Now the shoot begins to grow
Tall, taller, tall as can be,
The shoot is growing into a tree.
And branches grow and stretch and spread
With twigs and leaves above your head.
And on a windy autumn day
The nut tree bends, the branches sway,
the leaves fly off and whirl around,
And nuts go tumbling to the ground;
Small, brown, hard, round.
Julia Donaldson - Writer

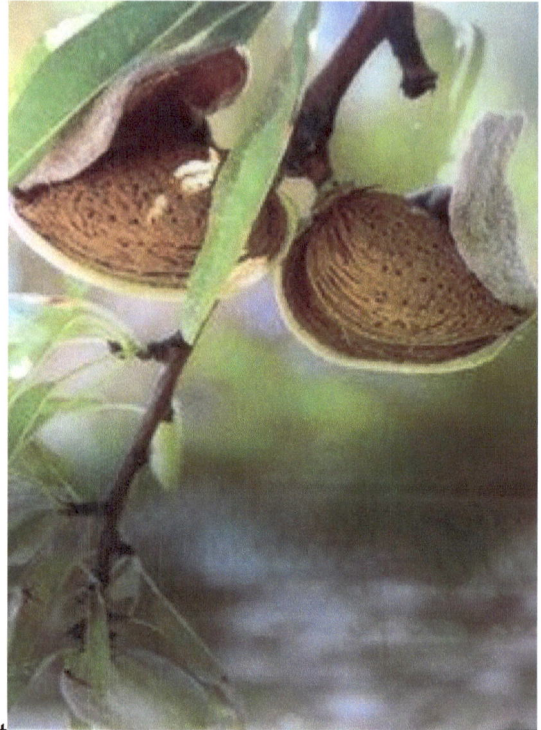

Nuts have been a favorite food since ancient times, and they have also been used as a medicine, as supported by the famous physician Hippocrates, who said nuts can help to cure many diseases. Nuts are a healthy and nutritious snack and are much better than chips and sweets. They reduce cardiovascular disease, strengthen the heart muscle, and prevent the development of diabetes. Lecithin, a fat found in nuts, improves memory. A handful (25 g) of nuts equals approximately 123-160 calories. As nuts are not easy to digest, they should be eaten in small quantities. They are best eaten unroasted and without added sugar or salt. Nuts can be stored in either a refrigerator or in a bag, and they will be fresh and tasty for about 3-4 months. The simplest foods are most often the best for your health, and this is certainly the case for nuts, in which Mother Nature has crafted a nearly perfect package of protein, healthy fats, fibers, antioxidants, and many vitamins and minerals.

Eating 30g nuts, 10g raisins, and 50g cheese every day helps to tone the central nervous system, eliminate the onset of fatigue and headaches, and strengthens the heart muscle.

ATTENTION. More and more people, especially children, are allergic to nuts, especially peanuts (which isn't actually a nut). If you are allergic to nuts, when in a restaurant or having dinner at a friend's house you should ask whether they are included in a dish.

Walnuts

Walnuts (Jupiter's nut). Walnuts belong to the tree nut family and are perhaps the oldest tree food known to man, dating back to 7000 B.C. The Romans called walnuts Juglans regia, which roughly translates as "Jupiter's royal acorn."

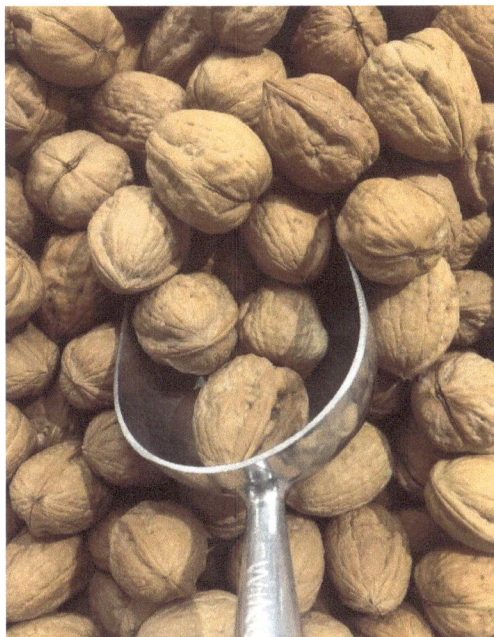

The history of early English walnuts suggests they came from ancient Persia, where they were reserved for royalty. Thus, the walnut is often known as the "Persian walnut."

Some consider the walnut to be king of all nuts, as research shows they can boost your health in a number of ways at very easy-to-achieve doses.

The first commercial planting of walnuts began in the US in 1867 in Santa Barbara County. California walnuts account for 99 percent of the commercial US supply and form three quarters of the world walnut trade.

Eating just one ounce of walnuts a day (about seven shelled nuts) is enough to take advantage of their beneficial properties.

Walnut Health Benefits

One-quart cup of walnuts (about one ounce) provides more than 100 percent of the daily recommended amount of omega-3 fats, along with a high amount of copper, manganese, molybdenum, and biota.

Some of the most exciting research about walnuts includes cancer-fighting properties, heart health, rare and powerful antioxidants, weight control, improved reproductive health in men, brain health, epilepsy, bone health, weight management, gallstones, thyroid diseases, and diabetes.

Recipe
For a nutritious breakfast, mix 2 teaspoons of crushed walnuts with 200 ml of plain yogurt. Add raisins and 1 teaspoon of honey.

Cashew

Cashew botanicals (Anacardium occidentale) are the seed of a tropical evergreen shrub related to the mango and the pistachio. They are native to South America and Brazil. Colonists first introduced the cashew to East Africa and India in the 16th century. These regions are now the largest producers of cashews.

Cashew nuts are one of the lowest-fiber nuts, packed with vitamins, minerals, and antioxidants that include vitamin E, K, and B6, as well as minerals such as copper, phosphorus, zinc, magnesium, iron, selenium, all of which are important for maintaining a healthy body. While high in fat, all nuts are ranked highly for their unsaturated fats. It is recommended to eat 6-7 cashew nuts a day.

Cashew Health Benefits

Cashew nuts have a number of benefits, including: Improved heart health, lower cholesterol, weight management, the prevention of cancer, a reduced risk of requiring a cholecystectomy if suffering from gallstones, and improved bone health. In addition, cashew nuts lower high blood pressure, maintain healthy nerves and a healthy head of hair, aid digestion, are high in vitamins, maintain healthy gums and teeth, reduce macular degeneration, and induce pleasant sleep.

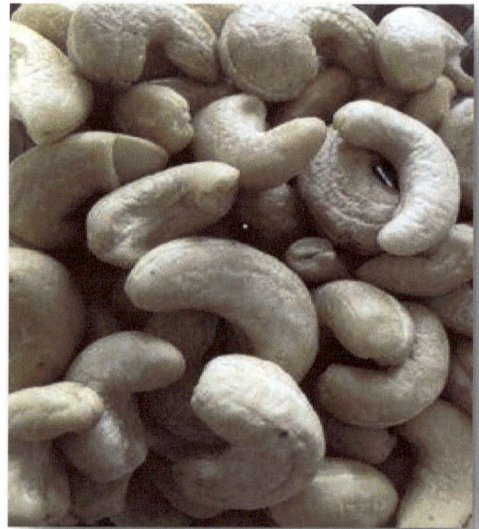

Almonds

Almonds (Prunus dulcis). Almonds are mentioned as far back in history as the Bible. They were a prized ingredient in the bread served to Egypt's pharaohs. Almonds are thought to have originated in China and Central Asia. The Romans considered almonds a fertility charm and gave them to newlyweds. There are more than 30 varieties of almonds. Many almond trees do not self-pollinate and depend on bees to carry pollen between them.

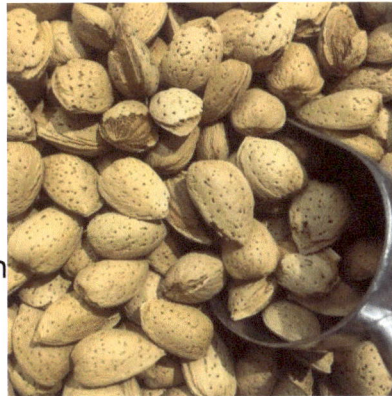

The United States—primarily California—produces 83 percent of the world's almonds, followed by Australia (7 percent), the European Union (5 percent), and Iran and Tunisia (all 1 percent). Almonds should be stored in cool, dry conditions away from direct sunlight, as well as away from any foods with strong odors, which almonds can absorb.

Almonds Health Benefits

Every one-ounce serving (about 23 almonds) contains all of our daily protein needs. Almonds provide 6 grams of protein fiber, plus vitamin E (35 percent daily value, DV), Magnesium (920 percent DV), riboflavin (20 percent DV), calcium (8 percent DV), and potassium (6 percent DV). Almonds are filled with minerals such as magnesium, copper, potassium, calcium, phosphorus, iron, and B vitamins. Almond has the lowest fat content of all the nuts.

The benefits of almonds: maintain a healthy heart, weight loss, and the prevention of weight gain, good for a gluten-free diet, prevents diabetes, a good source of energy, prevents gallstones and osteoporosis, lowers cholesterol, cancer-fighting properties.

Brazil nuts

Brazilian nut tree (Bertholletia excelsa). Brazil nuts are the only species in the monotypic genus Bertholletia. It is native to the Guianas, Colombia, Venezuela, Brazil, eastern Peru, and eastern Bolivia. Typically found as scattered trees in large forests on the banks of the Amazon River, the Rio Negro, the Tapajos, and the Orinoco. Brazilian nuts are an excellent source of B vitamins and minerals such as manganese, selenium, potassium, calcium, iron, phosphorus, and zinc. They also contain a low amount of vitamin E and are high in fiber.

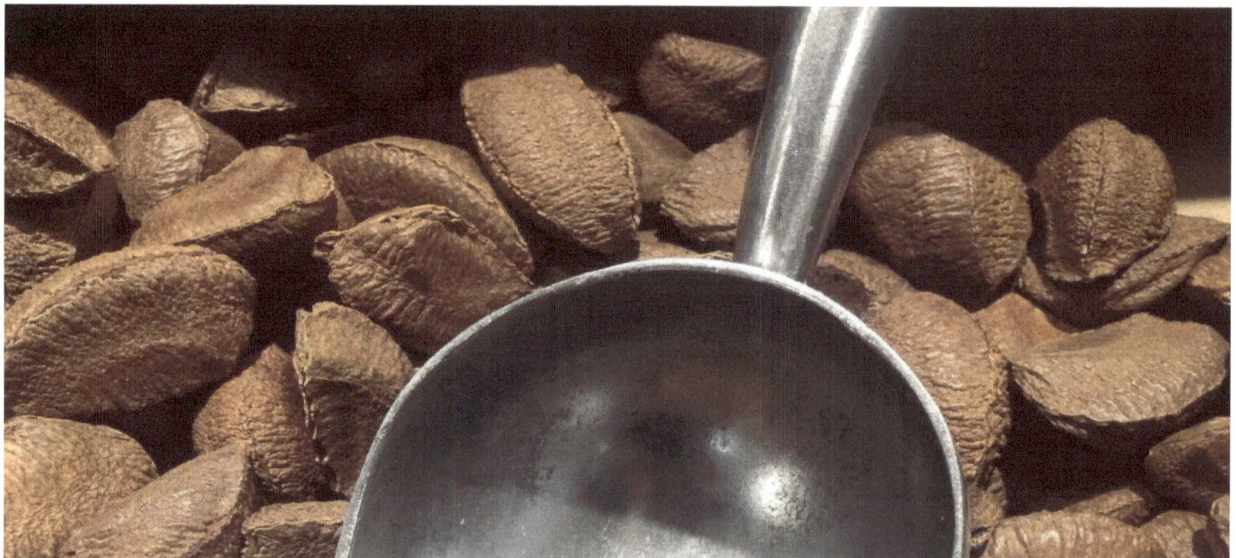

The Health Benefits of Brazil Nuts

Brazil nuts are an incredibly powerful antioxidant. They are high in fat and have a high calories content, though too many of them can lead to selenium toxicity. Eating just 2-3 nuts a day will supply you with a boost of vitamins, minerals, and nutrients.

Brazil nuts have more benefits, which include thyroid protection, improved mood, lower cholesterol, healthy hair and nails, and glowing firm skin. Brazil nuts also fight against breast cancer, acne, and psoriasis.

Pine nuts

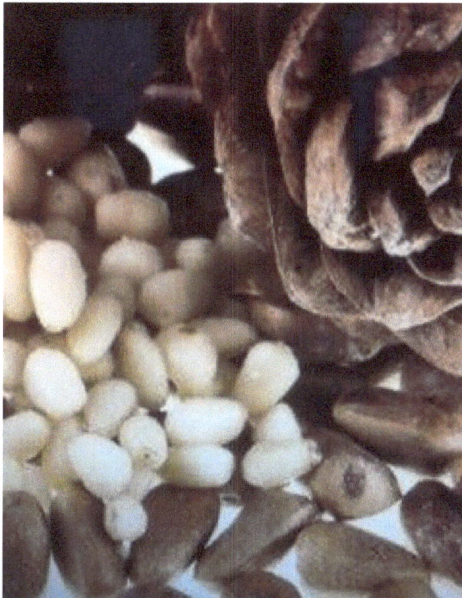

Pine nuts (pignoli) belong to the Pinaceae family. Pine nuts have been enjoyed since ancient times, even mentioned by Greek authors as early as 300 BC, and there's evidence that turn of millennium Roman soldiers ate them on campaigns.

Unshelled pine nuts are prone to rancidity due to their high oil content (so be sure to store them in your fridge). Afghanistan is an important source of pine nuts, though China and Korea are the main producers. Pine nuts produced in Europe mostly come from the stone pine (Pinus pinea), which has been cultivated for its nuts for over 5,000 years and harvested from wild trees for far longer.

Pine Nuts Health Benefits

Pine nuts contain heart-friendly monounsaturated fats and iron, both of which help the nervous system. They are a good source of protein and magnesium, which helps boost energy, while the vitamin D content builds stronger bones. In addition, vitamin C boosts the immune system, and anti-aging antioxidants and nutrients support the heart and maintain healthy vision. Pinolenic acid may also help weight loss.

It is recommended that humans eat about 100 pine nuts a day.

Hazelnuts

The hazelnut derives from the hazel, especially the nuts of the (Corylus avellana) species. It also is known as the cobnut or filbert nut, depending on the species. The original name was connected with Saint Philbert's Day on August 22nd (Saint Filbert), which is the name given to the hazelnuts and the tree in England when it was introduced by French settlers; however, the English later changed the name to hazelnuts.

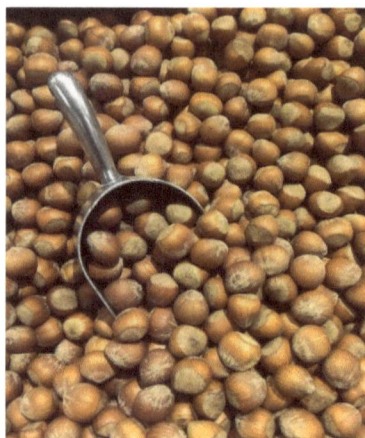

Today, the world's primary exporter of hazelnut come from the Black Sea region of Turkey, although they are also grown in the US Pacific Northwest and many other parts of the world.

In ancient times, hazelnuts were used as a medicine and a tonic, as mentioned in Chinese manuscripts that date as far back as 2838 BC. Hazelnuts bloom and pollinate in the middle of winter and are typically harvested in late September or October after they fall to the ground.

Hazelnuts Health Benefits

They are rich in saturated fats (mostly oleic acid), as well as magnesium, calcium, and vitamin B and E. It is recommended to eat a small handful a day, about 30 grams, which equals about 20 hazelnuts.

Hazelnuts promote heart health and help manage diabetes. They are also filled with antioxidants, boost the brain, help prevent cancer, combat obesity, and contribute to healthy skin and hair.

Pecan

Pecan (Carya illinoinensis). The pecan is a Native American word of Algonquin origin that was used to describe all nuts requiring a stone to crack. Originating in central and eastern North America and the River Valley of Mexico, the Native Americans taught the early colonists how to harvest, store, and utilize the pecan as an essential source of nourishment throughout the harsh winters. Today, the United States boasts a flexible pecan production flow that stretches across North and South Carolina, Arkansas, Oklahoma, Kansas, Texas, New Mexico, Arizona, and California.

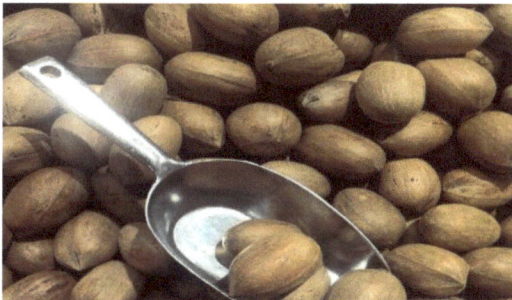

Pecan nuts are high in healthy unsaturated fats and can lower bad cholesterol. They also contain more than 19 vitamins, minerals, and vitamins including A, B, and E, folic acid, calcium, magnesium, phosphorus, potassium, and zinc.

It is recommended to eat about 8-9 pecan nuts a day.

Health Benefits of Pecan

Pecan nuts are good for the cardiovascular and digestive systems. They also reduce blood pressure, prevent strokes, and have anti-cancer properties. They strengthen the immune system, promote hair growth, prevent hair loss and skin problems, and have anti-aging benefits. Lastly, they aid weight loss, and promote bone and teeth health.

Pistachio

Pistachio (Pistacia vera). Pistachio nuts are one of the oldest nuts to be cultivated and consumed in the world. Recent archeological evidence from Turkey suggests that humans enjoyed pistachio nuts as early as 7,000 BC. Flourishing in hot climates, pistachios spread from the Middle East to the Mediterranean, quickly becoming a treasured delicacy among royalty, travelers, and common folk alike.

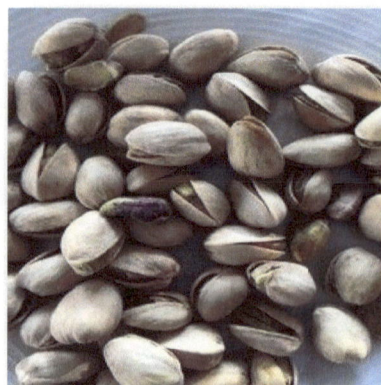

France is the largest producer of pistachios in the world.
The second largest is California, where 98 percent of pistachios produced in the US originate.

Health Benefits of Pistachios

Pistachio nuts contain 13 grams of fiber and 25 grams of high-quality of nutrients, such as thiamin, vitamin B6, copper, manganese, phosphorus, magnesium, and iron. The vitamins, minerals, fats, and proteins found in pistachios are all very good for your health. Just a half cup of shelled pistachios with no added salt has 170 calories, 13 grams of fat, and 1.5 grams of saturated fat.

Pistachios promote a healthy heart, help with weight management, and protect against diabetes and hypertension. They also improve digestion, eliminate skin dryness, contain dietary fibers, and have antioxidant properties. Further, pistachios nuts prevent the onset of age-related macular disease.

Pistachio nuts are a relatively low-calorie snack. It is best to use fresh and natural pistachio nuts, and eat about 15 a day.

Macadamia Nuts

The macadamia nut (macadamia) is a genus of four species of trees indigenous to Australia and constitute a part of the plant family Proteaceae. The nut is native to north eastern New South Wales and central and south eastern Queensland. Macadamia typically grow in tropical climates, such as Australia, Brazil, Indonesia, Kenya, New Zealand, and South Africa. Macadamia trees have also been planted in Hawaii. Macadamia trees can reach 40 feet in horizontal as well as vertical spread. California and Hawaii are now the world's largest exporters of Macadamia nuts. A tree that is 10-years-old might produce up to 50 pounds of Macadamia nuts a year.

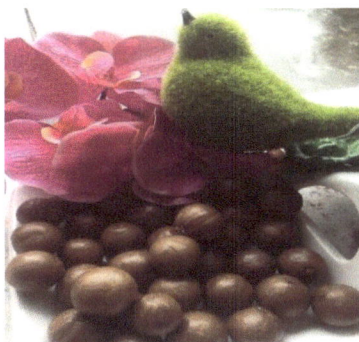

Macadamia nuts are a good source of vitamin A, E, B, iron, protein, thiamine, riboflavin, and niacin. They also contain a small amount of selenium (an antioxidant), calcium, phosphorus, potassium, and magnesium.

Health Benefits of Macadamia Nuts

Macadamia nuts are rich in fat and low in protein. Macadamia nut consumption should be limited because of their high-calorie content.

Macadamia nuts help to keep your heart healthy, fight free-radical damage, which leads to cancer, curb your appetite, strengthen your hair, skin, and nails, support gut health, strengthen bones, promote the brain and nervous system, and encourage weight loss.

Warning: Macadamia nuts are toxic for dogs, causing a non-fatal syndrome of vomiting, weakness, and neurological signs.

Chapter 8

GOD-GIVEN FOOD

In the middle...growing tree of life, yielding twelve fruits,
Leading fruit every month, tree leaves and is suitable to
treat the nations.
- The Blessed Sacrament, Rev. 22:2.

God has given us signs, and we do not even have to
read between the lines.

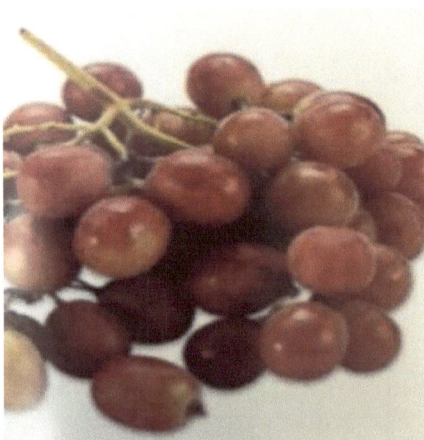

Grapes are heart-
shaped and look like
blood cells. Today's
research shows that
grapes have excellent regenerative properties for the
heart and blood.

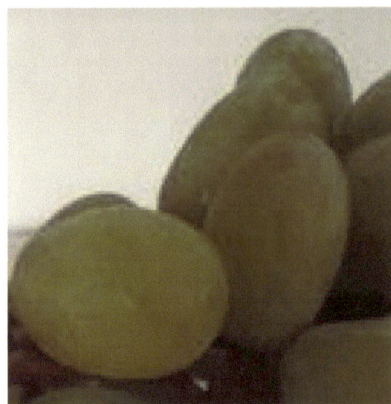

Citrus fruits are reminiscent of breast glands and
improve lymphatic circulation in breasts.

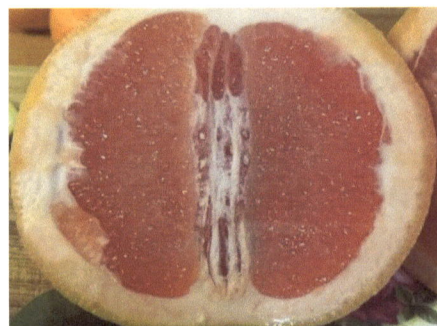

Figs are full of seeds and hang in pairs when they
are growing. Figs increase the capacity of male
sperm, while they also help to treat male infertility.

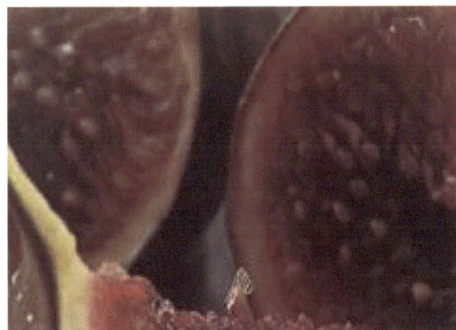

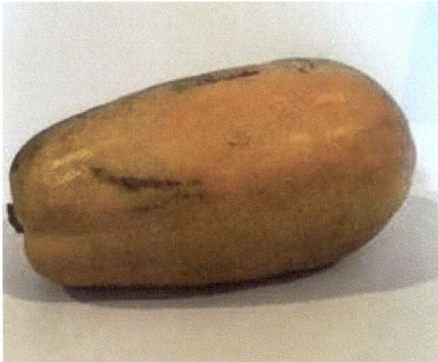

Eggplants, avocados, papaya and pears focus on the health and function of a woman's uterus and cervix, and they look just like these organs. Research shows that eating 1 avocado a week stabilizes hormones, increases weight loss, and prevents cervical cancers from developing. One suggestion is to choose mashed avocado over mayo. Spread the avocado on whole wheat bread, either alone or in a sandwich, to feel the benefits from the avocado's healthy fat, fiber, and vitamins.

Onions look like the cells of the body. Modern research shows that onions help to remove the toxins carried in all body cells. In addition, onions provoke the production of tears in humans, which clean the epithelial layers of the eyes.

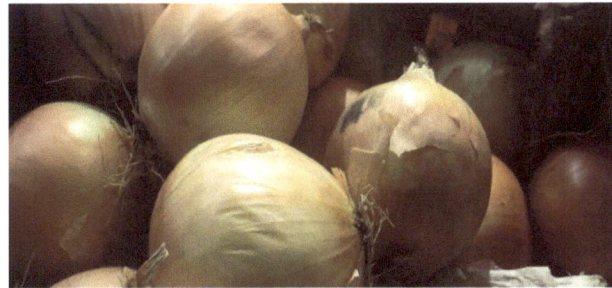

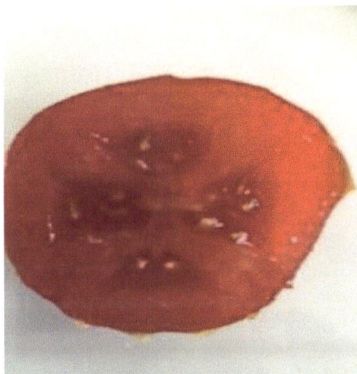

Tomatoes have four chambers and are red; likewise, the heart also is red and has four chambers. Prior research indicates that tomatoes are indeed a blood food.

At first glance, **celery, Chinese cabbage, and rhubarb** look like bones. This food adds strength to the bones, and these vegetables help to replenish the skeletal needs of the body.

Cut carrot looks like the human eye. Radiating lines look just like the human eye. Science now shows that carrots can greatly enhance blood flow and the function of the eye.

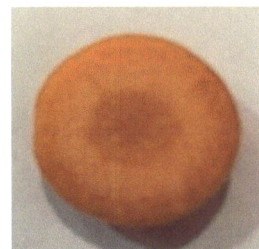

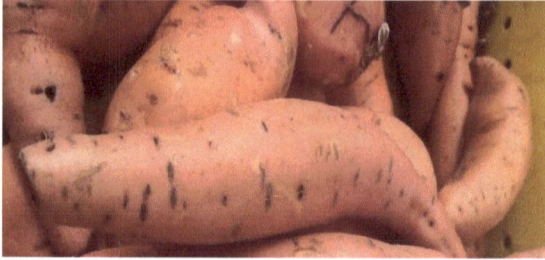

Sweet potatoes look like the pancreas and balance the glycemic index of diabetics.

Beans, shaped like kidneys, heal and help maintain healthy kidney functioning.

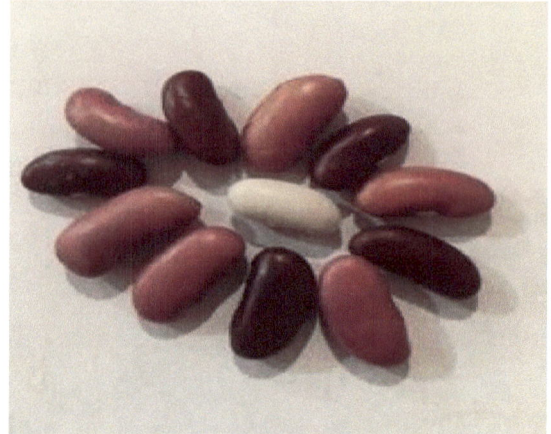

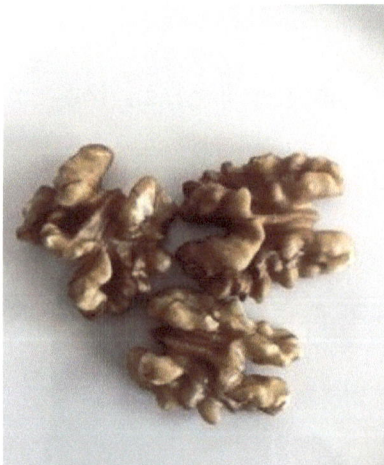

Walnuts look like a little brain—a left and right hemisphere, an upper cerebellum and a lower cerebellum. Even the wrinkles or folds on the nut look like the brain cortex. Walnuts help to develop more than 36 neuro-transmitters in the brain.

Olives improve the functioning of the ovaries and general health.

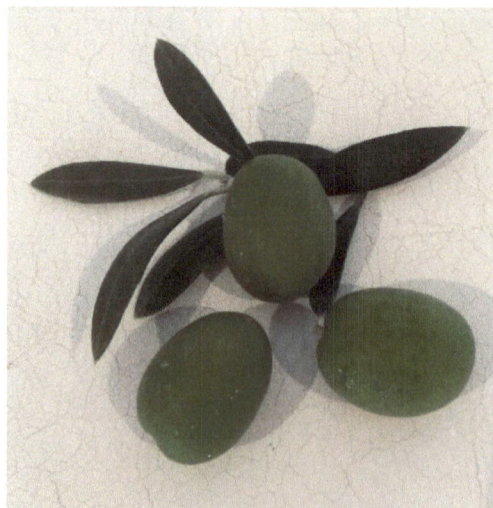

Chapter 9

CEREAL CROPS

It is only the farmer who faithfully plants seeds in the Spring who reaps a harvest in the Autumn.
--Bertie Charles Forbes, American author, Forbes magazine founder, 1880-1954

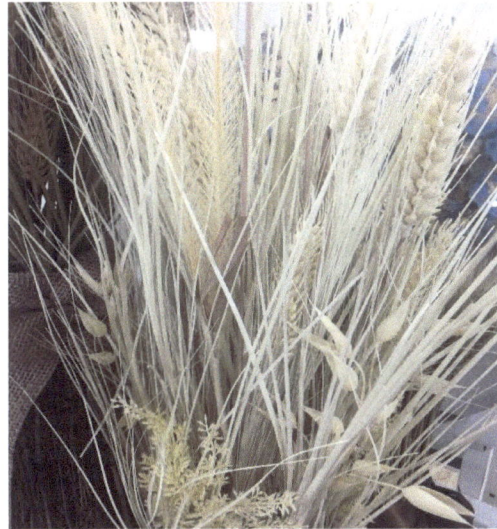

Grains are made from husked, crushed, or whole grains of various cereals, such as wheat, barley, buckwheat, and oats. They are rich in carbohydrates (about 50-70%), thus making them a major source of energy. Grains also contain a considerable amount of proteins (e.g., oat grains have up to 15% proteins, semolinas have up to 13.3%), fat (oats contain fat up to 7.8%, semolinas contain fat up to 1.4%), vitamins B1, B2, PP, E, various minerals, and they are also a great source of fiber.

By the end of the 19th century, grains were flushed with a hammer and then ground with handmade mills.

Traditional dishes made from buckwheat grain or flour were considered as commoner food, however, many of these dishes are biologically valuable and they are very much loved now.
Porridge is prepared from grain, and so too are baked pudding, flat cakes, pies, and pancakes. Before preparing the dishes, the grains are washed, and the small grains are sifted again.
Grain porridges should be boiled. Some prefer to cook them until they are completely dry, though others prefer leaving them thinner with more liquid content.

Dry grains are generally cooked from larger grains. Water is used most of the time, while water diluted with milk or broth is also typical. Buckwheat is usually soaked in broth or water in the evening before cooking so that it becomes swollen and boils faster in the morning. These grains are then poured into salted boiling water. If you prepare dry porridge, take 1 glass of grain and 2-2½ glasses of water or broth. Cook on a low heat. Stir until the grains are swollen, then cover. Finish cooking in the oven.

Thick porridges are boiled in water diluted with milk, and less often in water. Porridge is stirred constantly so that it will not burn. Take 1 glass of grains, 2-4 glasses of water (take 2 glasses for buckwheat grains, 3 glasses for rice, and 4 glasses for pellets).

Thin grain porridges are cooked in milk (or in milk with water). Take 1 glass of grain and 4-5 glasses of milk (or milk diluted with water).

Nobody doubts the **benefits of porridge oats**. By eating porridges and other meals from grains we get a minimum of 15 essential ingredients for the body: vitamins, minerals, carbohydrates, and vegetable fats.

Scientific research has shown that people who eat porridge in the morning eat less caloric and healthier snacks, so they find it easier to maintain a healthy weight and do not suffer from obesity. Porridge perfectly suits a full-fledged breakfast and reduces the tendency of over-eating during daytime, and especially in the evening.

Oats

Oats (Avena sativa). Oats are usually eaten like oatmeal porridge and are often used for baked wares such as oat biscuits. Oats are among the most useful foods for people. 100 g of oats contains 66.3 g of carbohydrates, which will give you enough energy to start your day. Oats provide a natural source of dietary fiber, which can help reduce the amount of bad cholesterol in our bodies. Oats contain a significant amount of B vitamins and are also a great source of minerals.

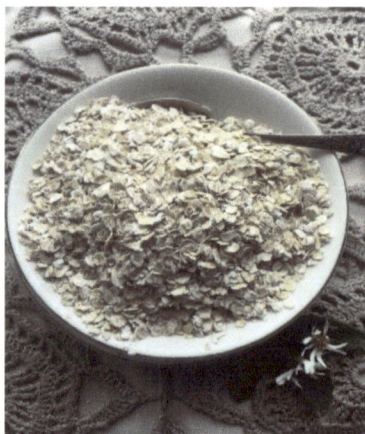

Health Benefits of Oats

Oats can reduce the risk of cardiovascular diseases. Harvard studies have shown that people who eat a bowl of uncrushed grains on a daily basis had a 20% lower risk of heart failure. The fibers in oats reduce cholesterol levels. Rich in beta-glucan, Oats protect the immune system against bacteria and microbes. Oats reduce the risk of cancer, reduce blood pressure, regulate blood sugar, and help with gastrointestinal disorders.

Recipes:

Oatmeal Porridge with Berries
Ingredients:

- 750 ml (3 cups) of water,
- 1 cup of oatmeal,
- 2 teaspoons of butter,
- a pinch of salt,
- 200g (5-6 tablespoons) of fresh or frozen berries.

Preparation: Boil water, add oat flakes to the water, salt, brew, and stir the porridge until it thickens. Remove from the heat, add some berries and stir the porridge. Pour into small bowls and decorate with the rest of the berries.

You can add a small piece of butter on the top of the porridge. Pouring sweet milk over your bowl of porridge oats can also liven up the recipe.

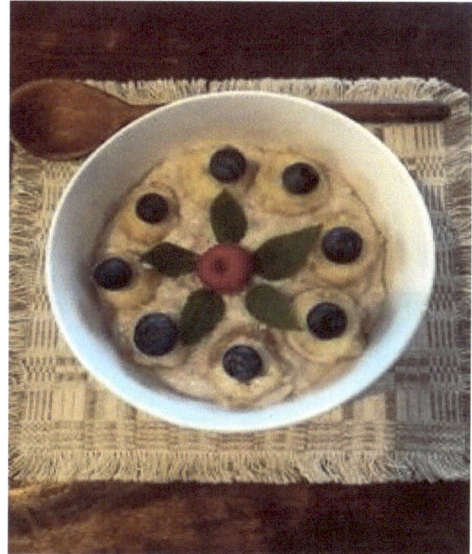

Oatmeal Cookies
Ingredients:

- 2 cups oatmeal,
- 2 cups all-purpose flour,
- 1 teaspoon baking soda,
- 1 cup unsalted butter at room temperature,
- 1 cup brown sugar, or less (to taste),
- 2 eggs,
- 1 teaspoon vanilla extract,
- 1/2 teaspoon cinnamon, 1/2 cloves, 1/2 nutmeg if desired,
- 2 tablespoons dried cranberries.

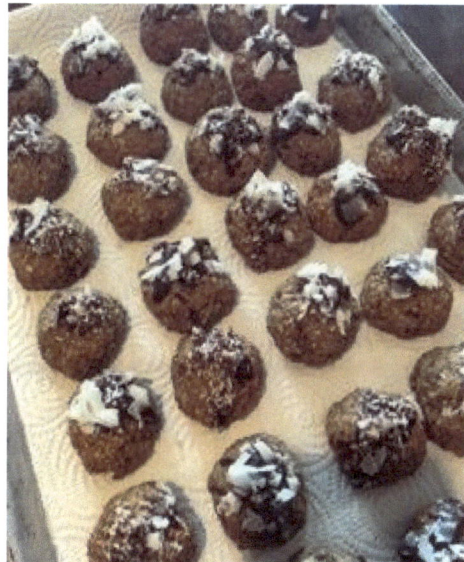

Preparation: Chop oats in food processor until fine, add flour and 1 teaspoon baking soda, mix together. To room temperature butter, add brown sugar and mix together until fluffy, add eggs and vanilla extract into the butter mixture, swirl until incorporated. Blend in flour mixture and cranberries. Spread butter on the baking tray to keep the cookies from sticking. Scoop the cookie dough out with a small ice-cream scoop, or by tablespoon, take in hands and roll into a ball. Place the cookies side by side on a baking tray and bake in a preheated oven at 350 degrees F (180 C) for 15-20 minutes until the oatmeal cookies become light brown. For extra decoration, consider adding chocolate drops or sprinkled coconut flakes. The oatmeal cookie dough can contain other ingredients, such as dried berries, fruits, nuts or sunflower or pumpkin seeds.

Flaxseed

Flaxseed (Linum usitatissimum). Flax is one of the oldest fibrous plants in the world. It grows mainly in Egypt, China, and in many European countries.

Health Benefits of Flaxseed

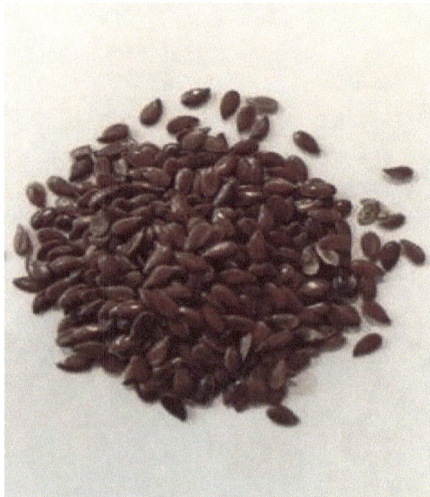

Flaxseed is a very valuable foodstuff with many important nutrients, including microelements, vitamin B1, fatty acids like Omega-3, and proteins. These acids inhibit the growth of cancerous cells and are useful for the heart, nervous system, and other body functions. Flaxseed also contains antioxidant substances and is one of the best sources of herbal hormone lignans. These are chemical compounds that reduce the risk of cancer, reduce cholesterol levels, and inhibit tumor growth. Flaxseed regulates blood sugar, protects against radiation and cancer, helps to regulate weight, strengthens immunity, reduces the likelihood of osteoporosis, and improves the functioning of the digestive system.

It is necessary to grind the flaxseeds in order for the body to better absorb them; if you eat whole seeds, they sometimes pass through the entire digestive tract and seeds are removed undigested.

Grind 2 tablespoons seeds with a coffee grinder and then pour ½ liter boiled water over them, allowing time for the water to be absorbed. Take this porridge (warmed) two times a day to treat constipation, one cup in a morning 30 minutes before breakfast and another cup at bedtime. The body best absorbs substances in this way. Flaxseed can be sprinkled on salads and added to yogurt, porridge, or pancakes.

It should be noted that pregnant women and people suffering from bowel obstruction **should avoid the consumption of flaxseed**.

Buckwheat

Buckwheat (Fagopyrum esculentum). The first buckwheat crops are thought to have been grown 8,000 years ago in Southeast China and the Himalayas when buckwheat was the main source of food for the local people. Later, buckwheat was replaced by rice and other grain crops. Buckwheat has many names. In India, it is called black rice; in France, Spain, and Belgium it is called Arabian grain, and in Greece and Italy, buckwheat is called Turkish grain.

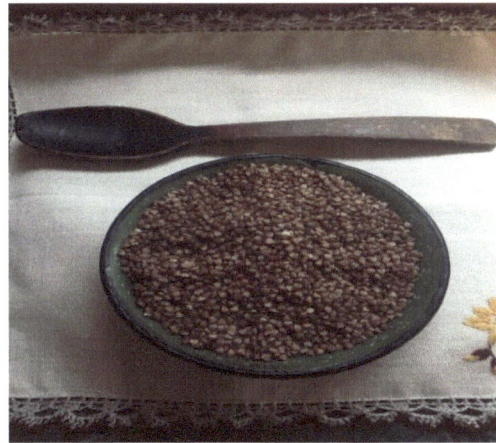

Health Benefits of Buckwheat

Buckwheat is a source of vitamin B, nutrients, and minerals.

There are 343 calories in 100 g of buckwheat. Buckwheat is a great source of energy. A good way to start your day is with buckwheat porridge.

Buckwheat improves digestion, helps to move food through the intestine, maintains intestinal cleanliness, thus preventing constipation. It also heals the liver, biliary disorders, and diabetes mellitus.

Buckwheat contains a large amount of folic acid, which stimulates blood flow and strengthens the body's resistance to adverse environmental influences. The high potassium and iron present in buckwheat prevent the body from absorbing radioactive isotopes and the formation of blood clots, in addition to reducing cholesterol.

Recipes:

Buckwheat Salad with Zucchini, Carrots and Feta Cheese
Ingredients:

- 100g (4 ounces) of buckwheat,
- 4 glasses of water,
- 1 medium-sized carrot,
- 1 zucchini,
- 1 clove of garlic,
- feta cheese,
- butter or oil.
- Spice per choice, such as a pinch of ground cumin, cilantro, turmeric, salt, black pepper,

Preparation: Rinse buckwheat with water two or three times and drain well. Soak the grains overnight in 4 glasses of water. In the morning, pour off the water.

In a frying pan, place butter or oil, add grated carrot and zucchini, and stir fry for 8 minutes. Add the buckwheat and spices and cook another 2-3 minutes. Transfer to a medium bowl, add feta cheese, and stir well.

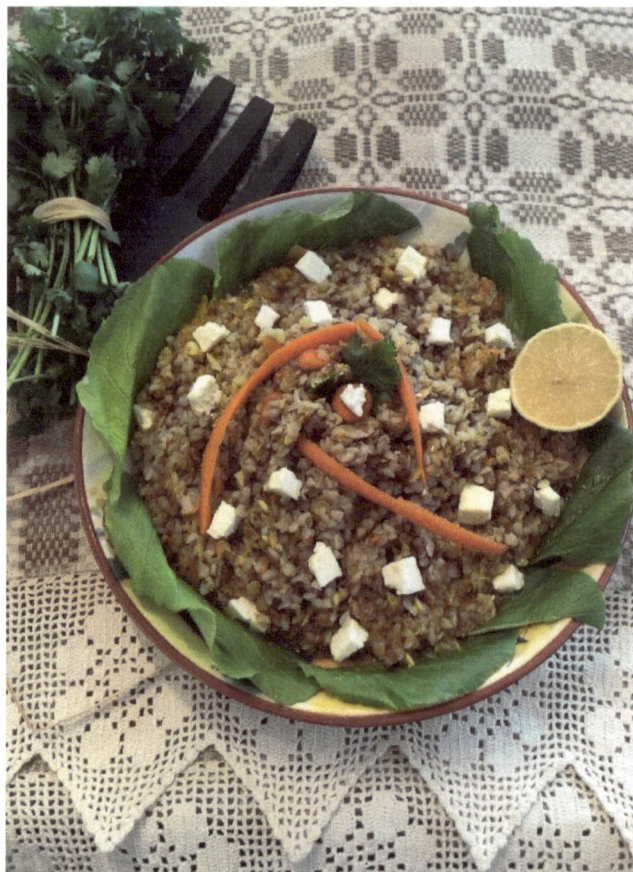

Buckwheat Porridge
Ingredients:

- 1.5 cups of buckwheat,
- 2 glass of milk
- 2 tablespoons of butter or olive oil, salt.
- Porridge fruits and nuts are excellent accompaniments to porridge, and you can also add a spoonful of butter or olive oil.

Preparation: Rinse buckwheat with water two or three times and drain well. Soak the grains overnight in 4 glasses of water. Add 2 glasses of milk, butter, and salt to a saucepan to boil. Add the buckwheat and boil over medium heat, stirring occasionally until mixture begins to thicken and the buckwheat has absorbed all the liquid. Cover, and allow to stand for 2-3 minutes.

Couscous

Couscous (Arabic kuskus). Couscous are small balls made of semolina, water, flour, and salt. Couscous originates from Maghreb, meaning "West" in Arabic. The region comprises three North African countries where Berbers used it as early as the 7th century: Tunisia, Algeria, and Morocco, as well as parts of Libya and Mauritania. It is the main wheat product of the Maghreb territory nations and a good source of carbohydrates. Couscous is sometimes referred to as "taam-food." The Arabs first brought it to France, and couscous soon became popular around the world. In the past, couscous was made manually and dried before the sun, but nowadays its production is automated.

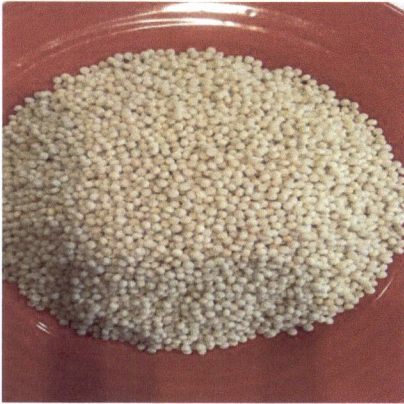

Health Benefits of Couscous

Couscous is a grain rich in carbohydrates. It is a major source of energy and rich in vitamins, minerals, vegetable fats, and proteins. Couscous is also a great source of fiber. All these useful nutrients help reduce the risk of cardiovascular diseases. Couscous regulates blood cholesterol, prevents many diseases, and treats constipation.

Small couscous grains are traditionally boiled in steam in a sieve hung above cooked meat or vegetables. Prepared couscous grains become clear, then they are carefully mixed with butter or other sauces and served as a garnish. They may be served as a side or an its own as a main dish.

Recipes:

Tabouli Couscous Salad

This salad originally came from the mountains of Syria and Lebanon. In Arabic, tabbouleh, or tabouli salad, is one of the main dishes. It became popular throughout the Middle East and has spread to other countries. It is a popular ethnic food in Western countries. Salads are eaten as a meal or as a garnish for various dishes, especially grilled ones. The main accent always must be a lot of parsley.

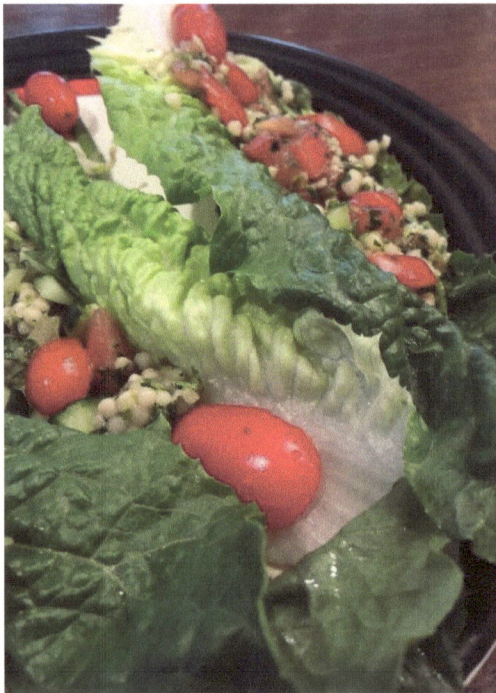

Ingredients:
- 125 g (4 oz) couscous,
- ½ cup of vegetable broth,
- ¼ tbsp of olive oil,
- ½ fresh lemon juice,
- 2 tomatoes,
- 1 onion,
- 2 small cucumbers,
- 1 bunch parsley leaves,
- 10 fresh mint leaves,
- Spices: ½ teaspoon cumin, ½ teaspoon of black pepper, salt.

Preparation: Put the couscous into a bowl and add boiling broth. Cover the bowl and soak for five - ten minutes until the grains become swollen. In a medium size bowl place sliced tomatoes, peeled and sliced cucumbers, finely chopped onion, fresh mint leaves, and chopped parsley. Pour drained couscous on top with sliced vegetables, add fresh lemon juice, olive oil, cumin, and black pepper. Mix thoroughly.

Chicken Salad

Ingredients:

- 150g (¾ cup) couscous,
- 1 glass of just-boiled water,
- 1 medium-sized carrot,
- 11-13 small-size mushrooms,
- 1 parsnip,
- 1 chicken breast fillet,
- 3 tablespoons of oil,
- 2 cloves of garlic,
- 1 cup of papaya,
- 2 tablespoons of sour cream,
- 2 tablespoons of lemon juice (lime if preferred).
- Spices: 1 chili pepper, salt, black pepper

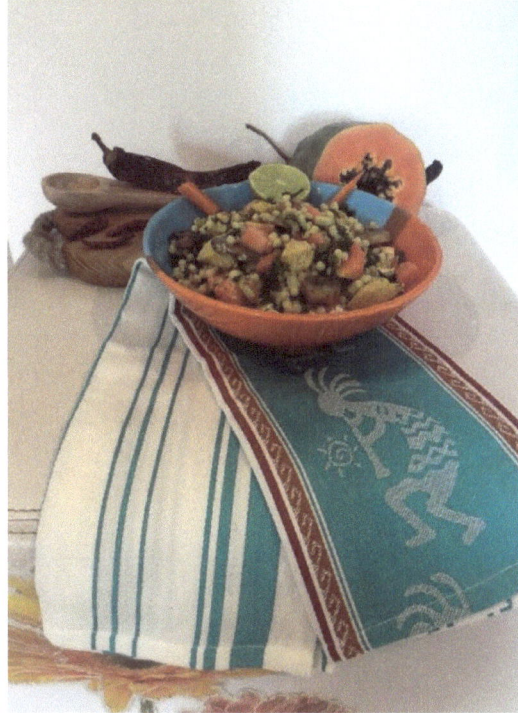

Preparation: Place the couscous in a pot, pour boiling water over it, cover, and leave to stand for five minutes. Cube or chop carrots and mushrooms. Cut the parsnips into slices, chop the garlic and take off the seeds from the chili peppers before finely chopping them. Once you have prepared the ingredients, add them to a pot with a small amount of water and stew. Cut the chicken into small pieces and add ½ cup of water to the pan. Boil for 2-3 minutes and remove the liquid. Once cooked, add the chicken to the stewed vegetables and stew together. At the end of the stewing, add the sour cream, couscous, peeled, seedless, and chopped papaya, lemon juice, salt, and pepper. Mix everything well. Top the salad with greeneries.

This dish can be eaten either warm or cold.

Couscous and Vegetable Salad

Ingredients:

- 150g (¾ cup) couscous,
- 1 glass of vegetable broth,
- 1 mango,
- 2 tablespoons of sugar cane sugar,
- 3 tablespoons of white wine vinegar,
- 3 small sweet onions,
- 1 clove of garlic,
- 3 tablespoons of oil,
- ginger slice,
- ½ yellow pepper, ½ red pepper, ½ green pepper,
- cedar or almond nuts,
- chili powder (according to taste).

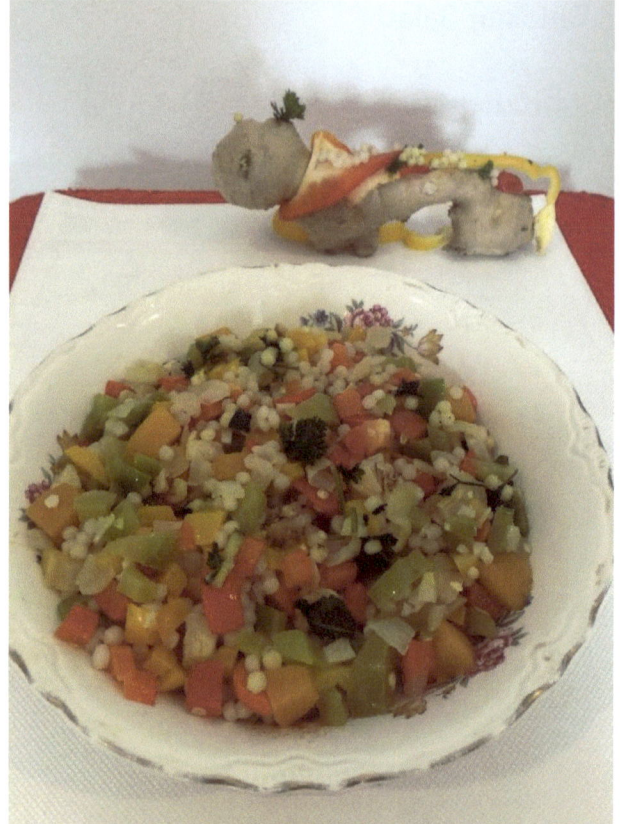

Preparation: Pour boiling broth over the couscous and cover for 5 minutes and remove from the heat, uncovered. Mix gently with a wooden spoon. Pour wine vinegar, oil, and sugar into a pan and mix it with a wooden spoon until the sugar dissolves. Add the sliced onion, garlic, and finely chopped ginger, pepper and stew. Finally, add couscous and sliced cubes of mango to the stew and stir.

Sprinkle the salad with cedar, almond nuts, or chili spice.

Quinoa

Quinoa (Chenopodium quinoa) is an herbaceous annual plant grown as a grain crop primarily for its edible seeds. Quinoa originated in the Andean region of northwestern South America and was domesticated 3.000 to 4.000 years ago for human consumption in the Lake Titicaca basin of Peru and Bolivia, though archaeological evidence shows livestock use 7000 years ago. Quinoa provides protein, dietary fiber, B vitamins, and dietary minerals in rich amounts above those of wheat, corn, rice or oats. It is gluten-free. Quinoa is an old plant used for food and cosmetics. Quinoa can be eaten as a hot porridge with spice or sweet porridge with milk (coconut, soy, almonds), yogurt, honey, nuts, or fruits and greens as a salad. Quinoa is an excellent addition to soups and stews. Like rice, it goes well with meat and fish. Some types of noodles and flour are also made from quinoa.

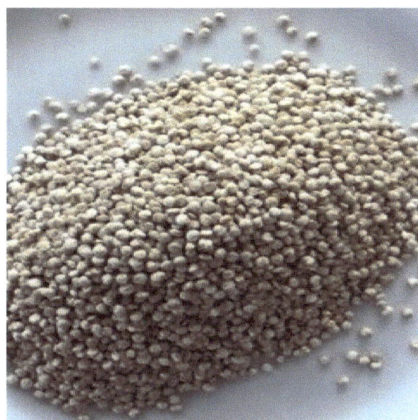

This plant does not belong to the cereal family, but its fruits are considered grains.

Health Benefits of Quinoa

Quinoa provides protein, dietary fiber, minerals, vitamins B, and vitamin E, low sugars, and saturated fat. In addition, the calcium and iron content are much higher in quinoa than in rice, corn, wheat, or oats. To increase the nutritional value of quinoa, it is best to sprout it for about 2-4 hours. Also, quinoa does not contain gluten, which can cause allergic reactions in some individuals. The nutritional value of quinoa per 100g is 356 kcal.

Recipe:
Quinoa is easy to prepare. First, rinse the seeds thoroughly in running cold water and then pour them into clean, cold, salted water. Mix 1 part of the grains with 2 parts of water or broth and cook on a medium heat and bring to boil. Reduce to a simmer for 10-15 minutes or until tender and the liquid absorbed. The boiled quinoa increases significantly and changes its shape as the grains become crispy.

Quinoa can substitute for oats in recipes. Boiled grains mixed with fruits, nuts, or honey form an excellent breakfast. Quinoa is often used in vegetarian dishes for its texture.

Quinoa and Parsley Salad

Ingredients:
- 1 ½ cups of water,
- ¾ cup of quinoa,
- ½ cup or less of lemon juice,
- 1 tablespoon of olive oil,
- ⅓ glass of thinly sliced parsley leaves,
- small cucumber,
- salt, pepper.

Preparation: Wash the quinoa well and boil. If there is still water left in the grains after boiling, filter it, add salt and pepper (according to taste), sliced cucumber, and parsley, and add it to the quinoa mixture. Mix everything. To garnish the dish, add a dash of lemon juice with olive oil over the top.

Cherry Walnut Quinoa Salad

Ingredients:
- 2 glasses of milk,
- 1 glass of quinoa,
- 1.5 glasses of halved and pitted (can also be frozen) cherries,
- ½ glass of walnuts,
- 4 tablespoons of liquid honey,
- ½ teaspoon of cinnamon,
- 3 tablespoons plain yogurt,
- ½ teaspoon chia seeds.

Preparation: Rinse the quinoa with water and boil with 2 glasses of milk. Reduce the heat and simmer for about 15 minutes or until tender. Put walnuts, cherries, and cinnamon with the boiled quinoa, let it cool a little bit, pour yogurt, add honey. Mix thoroughly, and top with sprinkled chia seeds.

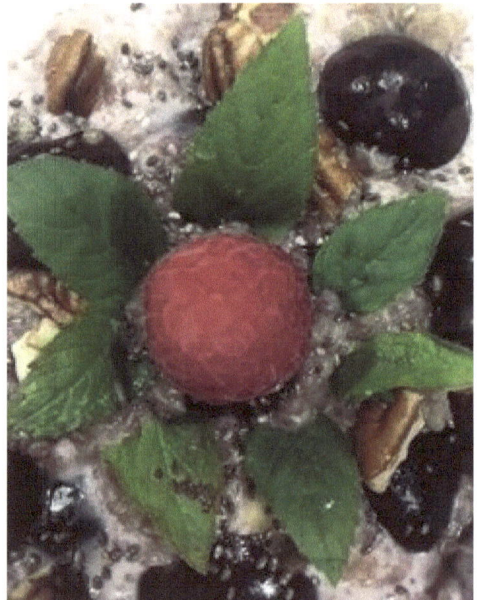

People who are allergic to honey, nuts, fruits, or other ingredients found in these grain dishes should **not eat** the salad.

Chapter 10

GELATIN, MILK (LACTIC ACID BACTERIA), AND YEAST

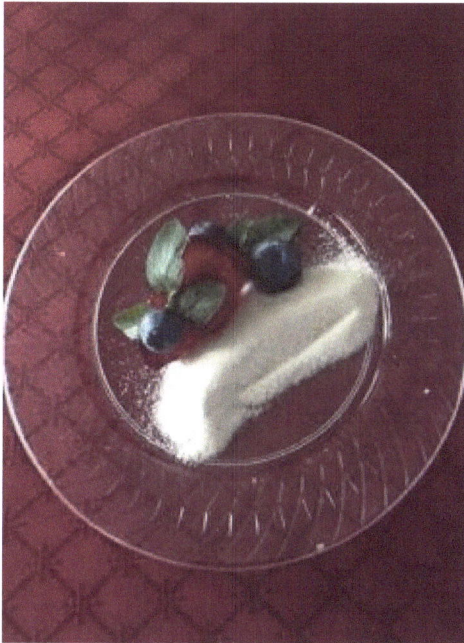

Gelatin

"The effects of gelatin are comparable to the collagen type 2 that comprises the connecting tissues in our body, counting the cartilage."
— Dr. Sundardas D. Annamalay.

Gelatin (gelato means stiff, frozen) is an animal protein mixture. Jelly is formed in water by boiling tendons, connective tissues, bones, skins, and other parts that contain collagen or proteins.

Pure gelatin is an amorphous, colorless, and shiny substance without taste or smell. It consists mostly of glycine and proline, which are amino acids used in collagen production.

100 g of gelatin contains 65.30 g of protein, as well as the following physiologically active micro elements: magnesium, sodium, potassium, calcium, iodine, and selenium.

When people learned to make pots of clay and cooked their first soups in ancient times, they realized that this jelly-like type of food was easily absorbed when eaten. Therefore, in ancient times, children, the sick, and the weak would typically be fed jelly.

Health Benefits of Gelatin

Jelly does not take but rather holds moisture and it is especially important for those with aging bodies, those who follow special diets, those who face high physical and nervous loads, and during hot spells when the body evaporates a lot of fluids.

In the human body, collagen contains a quarter of the body's required protein content. Over time, as people age, the skin wrinkles, the elasticity of the bones, ligaments, and joints decreases, the cartilage dissolves, the nails break up, and the hair shrinks. These effects can be slowed by consuming collagen from meat jelly, fish jelly, and gelatin.

Gelatin use improves the condition of the joints and reduces the inflammatory processes of the body. It combats arthritis and reduces inflammation after joint injuries. Anyone with arthritis or osteoporosis should use gelatin, which reduces joint pain and strengthens bones.

Eating jelly or gelatin will not cause you to gain weight as there is no fat or cholesterol content; on the contrary, its consumption encourages a graceful and straight posture. Breasts become firmer, cellulite disappears, and nails and hair become beautiful, strong, and shiny.

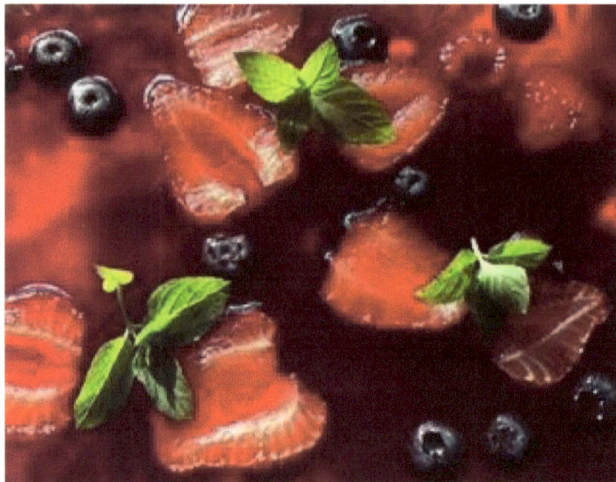

Wrinkles occur when the skin loses collagen, an effect that can be countered by consuming the amino acids found in gelatin. Athletes use collagen to help their bodies to recover from injuries.

Gelatin is useful to treat diabetes, blood disorders, and muscle weakness. It also benefits the intestines and improves digestion.

In gastronomy, gelatin is used to prepare a wide range of festive dishes that include vegetables, fish, poultry and meat, drinks, berries, and fruit desserts. Gelatin is recommended for those who cannot eat meat in their diets—jelly can be eaten without any restrictions. It is better to avoid chemically synthesized jelly, which increases cholesterol. Instead of consuming fat-storing pastries, cakes, and chemically synthesized ice cream from stores, make your own colorful and delicious jellies with berries, fruits, and vegetables.

To add color to the gelatin, add fresh berries and fruits. Cut the fruit into small pieces for better cohesion of the gelatin. Avoid using pineapples, papaya, or kiwi, as these contain enzymes that liquify the gelatin.

Physiologist Sean McCarthy of the Rippe Lifestyle Institute, Massachusetts, asked 175 elderly patients to drink a daily dose of 10 g of gelatin powder and compared it with a control group who did not use gelatin. Patients who took gelatin showed stunning results: they became stronger and performed better on physical exercises, particularly in those involving the knee joint. McCarthy believes that gelatin can maintain healthy cartilage, slowing or arresting its decay.

Development, Preservation, and Restoration of Human Connective Tissue

Add two teaspoons (about 10 g) of gelatin in a quarter cup of ice-cold water in the evening, stir, and leave overnight. In the morning drink the resultant gelatin with juice or warm, sweetened water before a meal. Within a week you'll find relief from pain in your legs, neck, and back. Drink this mixture for 21 days once a year. This is a natural way to restore joints; a "lubricant remedy", and many other organs work better when joints function normally. The autumn is a great time to use fresh berries, fruits, and vegetables in jellies to restore the vitamins and collagen in the body.

Gelatin test: Your gelatin should dissolve in cold water. If not soluble, throw it away.

Recipe:
Farmer's Fresh Cheese and Berry Cake with Gelatin

Fresh, or frozen berries are perfect for this colorful dessert. If you add a lot of blueberries, you will produce a strong, violet-colored dessert, or if you put a lot of cherries, currants, or strawberries, you will create cakes of different colors.

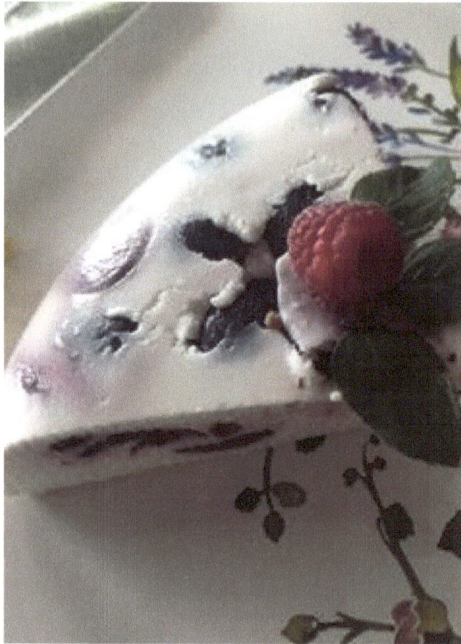

Ingredients:
- 360 g (1½ cup) farmer's cheese or cream cheese
- 300 ml. yogurt (better plain),
- 2 cups cherries without pits,
- 4-5 tablespoons sugar,
- 1 cup cold water to absorb gelatin,
- 1 teaspoon vanilla extract or vanilla sugar,
- 4-5 tablespoons gelatin,
- 1 cup water.

Preparation: Pour the gelatin in cold water, stir, and keep it for about 15 minutes until absorbed. Heat the water, then pour the absorbed gelatin in the pot and mix for about 1 minute until the gelatin dissolves. Leave until gelatin cools.

Mash the farmer's cheese with vanilla, add it to a manual blender or a food processor with the sugar and cherries. Add the dissolved gelatin and mix thoroughly. Pour the mass into a ready-made vessel and place in the refrigerator overnight. On the top of the dessert, you can lay out apricot halves, other fresh fruits, or even chocolate.

Milk

"The cow is of the bovine ilk; One end is moo, the other milk."
— Ogden Nash, American poet, 1902-1971.

Health Benefits of Milk

According to the National Dairy Council, milk contains nine essential nutrients that benefit our health. The three major nutrients in milk are calcium, which builds and maintains healthy bones and teeth; protein, which serves as a source of energy; and potassium, which helps and maintains a healthy blood pressure.

Yogurt

There is no precise date as to when yogurt was first created, but historical sources indicate that it was the favorite food of the Mongol conqueror Genghis Khan and his army in the 13th century. Yogurt has been widely used in the Middle East, Russia, and Bulgaria for centuries, although its benefits were only proven in the 20th century when lactic acid bacteria were found. Recently, the popularity of yogurt is growing worldwide, especially in the USA, Turkey, India, and Greece.

Yogurt can protect against many diseases. It improves the digestive system and helps obese people to adjust their weight. Yogurt contains iodine, calcium, potassium, phosphorus, the vitamins B2 and B12, protein, and zinc, as well as very useful probiotics.

Health Benefits of Yogurt

Live yogurt bacteria (lactobacillus acidophilus). Yogurt contains good bacteria that improve the intestinal microflora. Good digestion and a healthy digestive tract depend on these bacteria. These live and active cultures can protect against a range of bowel disorders, including colon cancer, irritable bowel syndrome, constipation, diarrhea, and lactose intolerance. Yogurt also helps to reduce cholesterol levels. All these benefits can be derived from as little as 200 ml of yogurt a day.

Many lactose-intolerant people enjoy yogurt because it does not induce digestive problems. According to scientists at the University of Tennessee, yogurt stimulates fat burning. Studies have shown that individuals who eat 85-170g of yogurt every day for 12 weeks burned twice as much fat as those who did not change their diet. The group which consumed yogurt enriched in probiotics and calcium supplements lost 22% more weight and 61% more body fat.

Yogurt also reduces the risk of cancer. A large-scale study of 45,000 volunteers, published in the International Journal of Cancer, showed that the use of yogurt can protect against colon and rectal cancer. This is because of the presence of probiotics and the good bacteria in yogurt.

Yogurt is high in potassium, which lowers blood pressure. Doctor of Medicine and Professor Alvaro Alonso at Harvard Public Health School conducted a study that found those who ate two or more portions of skimmed milk products had a 50% lower risk of increased blood pressure. Yogurt improves mouth odor, cleans plaque, and protects gum from diseases. Scientists say that human mood is directly related to intestinal health.

Use only natural yogurt without additives; yogurts that contain a large amount of sugar should be avoided as they promote caries.

Recipe:
Homemade Yogurt

Ingredients:
- 1 liter (1000 ml) of whole or 2% fat milk,
- 2 tablespoons of natural yogurt,
- thermometer.

Preparation: Boil milk on medium or low heat until bubbles appear in the hollow and vapors start to come out of the surface. Pour the heated milk into a large bowl and cool to about 45°C (113°F). If you do not have a thermometer, do it as the Greeks do (the temperature is perfect if you can hold the index finger in the yogurt for 20 seconds). Place the yogurt in a small bowl, add a little warm milk, and mix well. Add the resulting mixture back into the bowl one third at a time, stirring each portion thoroughly after each pouring. Cover with a thick cloth and keep it warm for 6-8 hours or overnight. If you keep yogurt for a shorter time, it will be sweeter, whereas if you keep it for a longer time, it will be more acidic. Once the yogurt has settled down, cover the bowl with cellophane and keep it in the refrigerator for several hours before eating. You can store yogurt for about 2 weeks in the refrigerator.

Farmer Cheese

"The king's cheese is half wasted in pourings, but no matter, 'tis made of the people's milk"
– Benjamin Franklin, 1706-1790.

Ingredients:
- 1 liter (1000 ml) of whole or 2% fat milk,
- 1 liter (1000 ml) of kefir or 1 liter (1000 ml) of yogurt.

Preparation: Heat the milk at high temperature but do not boil. Next, pour cold kefir or yogurt which will set the milk immediately. Then, put the mass into a colander and put a gauze in it, or put in a cheesecloth bag. If you want to have sweet farmer's cheese, add more milk. Hang the bag over the bowl and strain off.

Do not throw the whey away; keep it for pancakes or blinis.

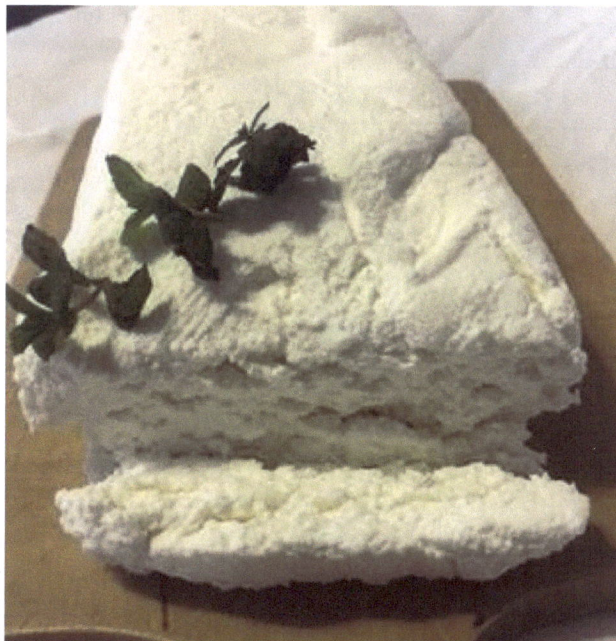

Ingredients:
- 1 liter of milk,
- ½ tbsp of lemon juice.

Preparation: Put the milk into a pot, heat it at high temperature but do not boil. After removing the pot from the hot surface, add lemon juice and stir. The milk should set and a greenish whey will be produced. If it was not successful, add more lemon acid. Put the mass in a gauze bag and leave to cool and dry. These quantities of ingredients should produce about 200 g of dry farmer's cheese.

Kefir

Kefir originated in the mountains of the northern Caucasus. Due to its bacteriological composition, kefir helps to regulate intestinal microflora, as well as digestive processes. Kefir helps to absorb nutrients while removing accumulated toxins from the body. Kefir provides vitamins A and B, as well as minerals, iodine, calcium, iron, and other useful substances for the individual. The bacteria found in kefir gives it a characteristic taste.

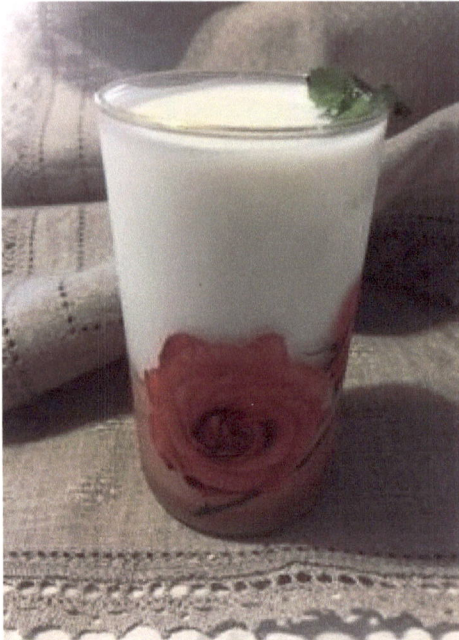

Health Benefits of Kefir

Kefir improves the appetite and stimulates gastric and intestinal peristalsis.

Kefir is recommended if you suffer from obesity, diabetes, liver and pancreatic diseases, gastritis (with decreased gastric acidity), or enterocolitis.

Constipation. To avoid constipation, drink 2-3 glasses of kefir per day.

Diabetes. Half an hour before breakfast and dinner, drink 1 glass of kefir mixed with 1-1.5 tablespoon of buckwheat flour (grind the buckwheat in a coffee grinder). The mixture should be made 7 to 8 hours before in order better to absorb it.

Osteoporosis. If you suffer from osteoporosis, a regular intake of kefir, buttermilk, farmer's cheese and other cheeses, and yogurt are recommended. There is a lot of calcium in fish, especially salmon, vegetable food, soybeans, sunflower seeds and sesame seeds, nuts, spinach, onions, and parsley. Not only should you try to eat foods containing calcium, but also foods containing magnesium and vitamin D. An abundance of magnesium is found in pineapples, bananas, parsley, dill, and potatoes (especially fried), while vitamin D is rich in fish and produced by direct sunlight. If you feel tired, it is advisable to drink a glass of kefir. It will help the body recover. The benefits of kefir also come in the fight against insomnia or nervousness. This drink improves memory, so it should be used by people working in mental occupations.

Skin. If you drink kefir regularly, your skin will develop a healthy glow.

If the flavor of kefir doesn't appeal to you, try adding flavorings:

1. In a glass of kefir, add 2 teaspoons of strawberry or cherry jam and mix well. Alternatively, add fresh berries.
2. In the warm summer season, prepare an excellent kefir drink by mixing equal parts of kefir and mineral water.
3. Drink 1 glass of kefir with boiled, still warm, fresh potatoes with sprinkled dill on them. A great, refreshing summer meal.

Yeast

"God made yeast, as well as dough, and loves fermentation just as dearly as he loves vegetation."
— Ralph Waldo Emerson, 1803-1882.

Yeast (Saccharomyces cerevisiae). Food yeast is a secret of good health. Yeast is mentioned in the oldest Egyptian medical document—the so-called Ebers papyrus, which suggests using yeast as an antidepressant drug. The Hippocrates followers and doctors in medieval monasteries used yeast as a natural remedy for high fever and diarrhea. In Persia and Arabia, yeast was an most important medicine due to the research of the famous Persian physician Avicenna.

Scientists have discovered that yeast stimulates the immune system, noting that its large amount of Vitamin B and minerals have antiviral and antibacterial properties.

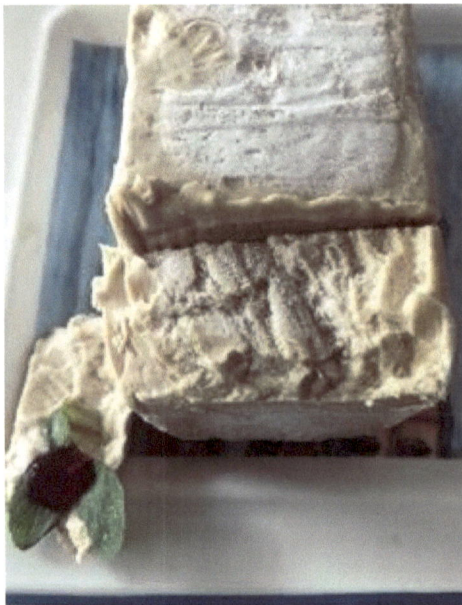

Food yeast and beer yeast belong to the same type of yeast. As beer yeast is very bitter, it is usually sold in capsules. The food yeast flavor is pleasant and is similar to cheese or nuts.

Food yeast can be found in health food stores. Yeast generally comes in the form of dry and loose flakes or granules. Thus, it worth adding 5-10 g to your daily diet or if in granules, 2 tablespoons of yeast-derived protein per day.

Health Benefits of Yeast

Food yeast can help when suffering from acne, decreased appetite (or if you desire to lose weight), disturbed digestion, diarrhea, or a fungal candida infection. Yeast stimulates the immune system, increases muscle mass, strengthens the hair and nails, and improves the condition of the skin. It is an energy-giving food that strengthens the body's resistance after exercise. At home, yeast should be stored in a dark and cool place, where it can be suitable for consumption up to 2 years. Food yeast can be used as a dressing for salads, soups, and stews, and can also be added to cocktails or cereals, giving a pleasant aroma to an array of dishes.

Using yeast cells, Dr. Lee Hartwell, a researcher from the US, investigated the processes of cell division of the human body. In 2001, he received the Nobel Prize of Medicine for his efforts. Dr. Feodor Lynen succeeded in isolating an important component of metabolism, the coenzyme A, from the yeast cell. For this study, which took place in 1964, Feodor Lynen received the Nobel Prize for Medicine. Ewald Dorling of Hamburg University tested enzyme yeast cell preparation on a group of athletes. The researcher found that preparation increased the body's resistance to physical, chemical, and biological stimuli, which increased the body's vitality. A number of studies from Japan have shown that glucans significantly reduce the mortality of cancer due to infection. The studies have confirmed that beta-glucans protect against bacterial infections, inflammation, and arterial sclerosis. Yeast beta-glucans can protect against infection before and after surgery; therefore, the use of enzyme yeast cells can reduce the need for antibiotics.

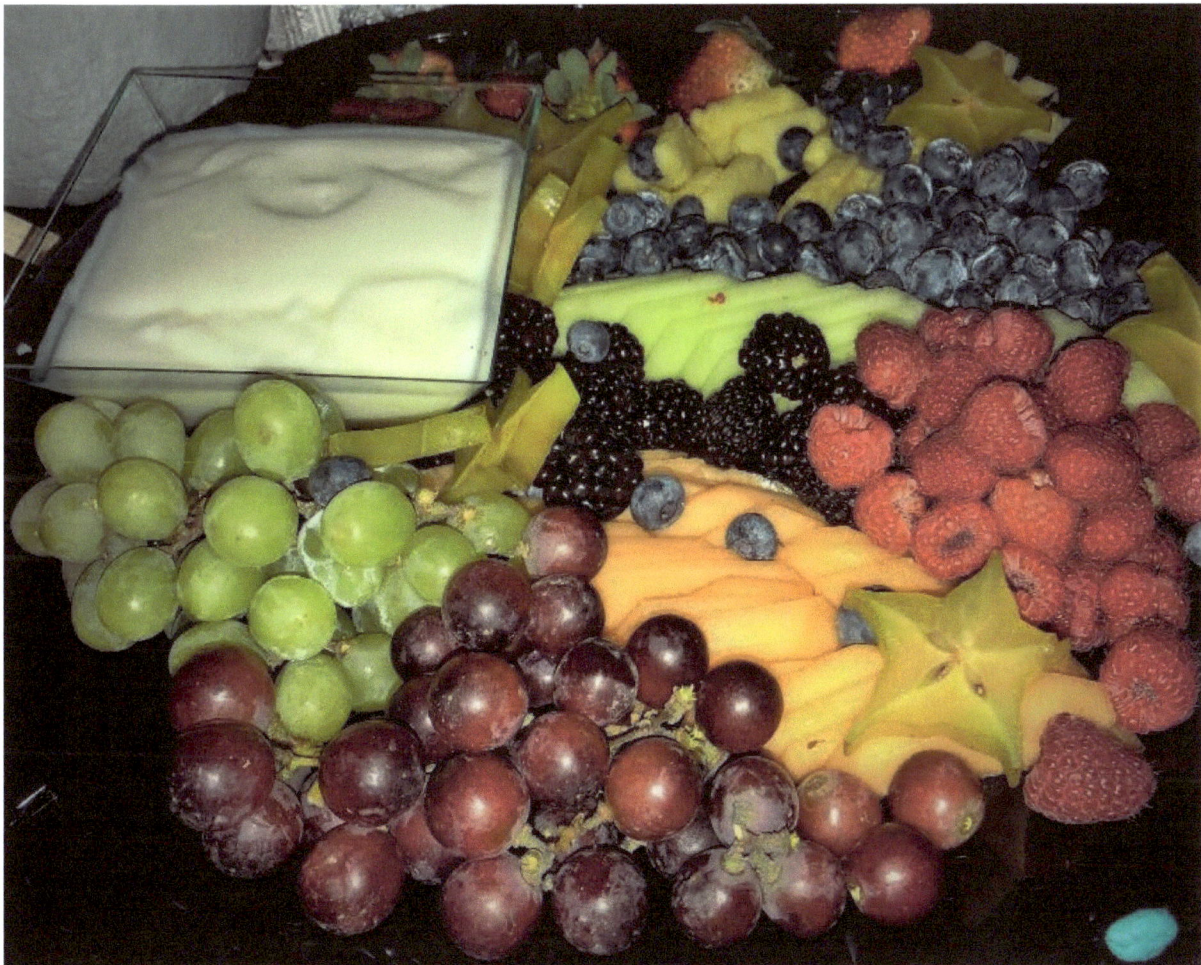

Chapter 11

TEAS AND THEIR USE

The essence of the tea ceremony–inside the participating communication, concentration, contemplation, conversation with oneself, with the arts and to respect the four fundamental principles of the tea ceremony–harmony, respect, purity, and tranquility.
– Romualdas Neimantas, Traveler and Writer.

Tea is the most commonly used beverage after water. In the Middle East, tea has been a source of good health, happiness, and wisdom for thousands of years. The main types of tea are green, black, white, and red. The green, black, and white teas are extracted from *Camellia sinensis* originating in China and India and red tea is extracted from *Aspalathus linearis*. The methods of their treatment and preparation different. The *Camellia sinensis* plant has a large amount of polyphenols, powerful antioxidants that include flavonoids that protect against the harmful effects of free radicals. These help prevent heart disease, cancer, and clogged arteries. The white tea is famous for this effect because it is the least processed of all teas.

Tea contains caffeine and theine, which stimulate mental alertness.

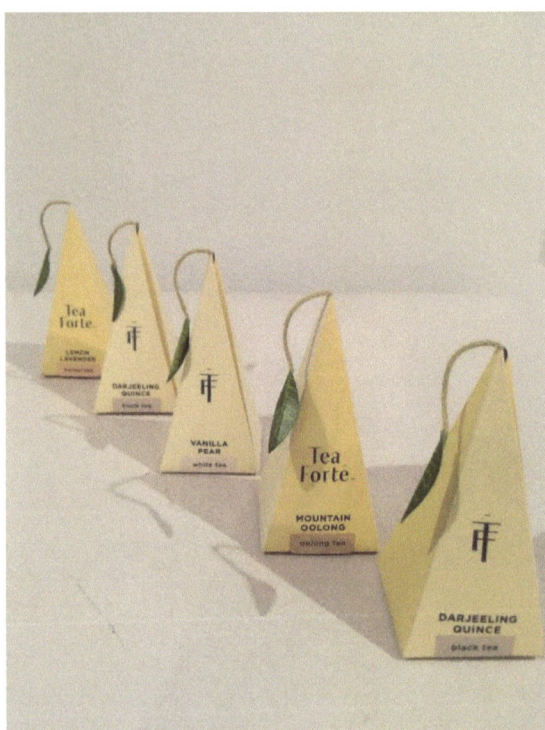

Green Tea. Green tea, made from *Camellia sinensis* leaves, is similar to Oolong tea, which is a deeper color green. However, green teas have not undergone the same withering and oxidation process used to make oolong teas and black teas. Green tea is produced by first evaporating or roasting the dried leaves and then re-drying them.

Health benefits of green tea: Green tea antioxidants can help with the prevention and progression of bladder, lung, stomach, pancreatic, and colon cancers. It helps to prevent blocked arteries by burning fat and reducing the risk of neurological diseases such as Parkinson's and Alzheimer's diseases. Green tea reduces the risk of strokes and has a positive effect on the cholesterol levels in the blood vessels. Green tea is best to drink after a meal.

Green Tea warnings. It may increase the risk of miscarriage for those drinking more than two cups per day. Green tea reduces iron absorption, so should be avoided in iron-deficiency. It increases the acidity of the stomach. The National Cancer Institute recommends consuming tea between meals. Caffeine in green tea might increase the risk of bleeding, irregular heartbeat, or anxiety. It may raise sugar levels in the blood if you suffer from diabetes, and for those with osteoporosis, green tea may stimulate the removal of calcium from the body. The Canadian Health Department warned that green tea has been associated with some liver diseases.

Black Tea. Black tea is made from fermented *Camellia sinensis* leaves. It contains the greatest amount of caffeine of all teas. Black tea contains antioxidants properties. Black tea may protect the lungs from the negative effects of smoking cigarettes, may lower the amount of bad cholesterol, boost heart health, improve gut health, reduce blood sugar levels, and reduce the risk of stroke.

White Tea. White tea is made from new growth buds and young leaves of the plant *Camellia sinensis*. The leaves are steamed or fried to inactivate oxidation and then dried. White tea is the least processed of all teas and has the most antioxidants.

Health benefits of white tea: It boosts cardiovascular health aiding to lower cholesterol, abates the risk of cancer, enhances weight loss, helps protect teeth from bacteria, and prevents certain nerve diseases. It may protect against osteoporosis, Alzheimer's, and Parkinson's diseases.

Red Tea. Red tea normally refers to rooibos tea. It is made using leaves from a shrub called *Aspalathus linearis*, a plant found only in the Cederberg Mountains on the western coast of South Africa. Traditional rooibos is created by fermenting leaves, which turn them a red-brown color. Rooibos tea is also known as red tea and red bush tea. South African mothers found that the tea soothed their babies' colic.

Health benefits of red tea: Red tea is packed with antioxidants, which reduces the risk of heart disease and reduces certain cancer risks. It may benefit those with type 2 diabetes, benefits bone health, improves digestion, and reduces allergies, headaches, and colic. While many of these claims have not been proven scientifically, researchers have established that it does promote the production of antibodies and delays the recurrence of the herpes simplex virus. A 2005 study found that rooibos protected against the growth of lesions associated with skin cancer. A similar study in 2008 conducted by Dr. Jeanine Marnewick of Cape Peninsula University of Technology (CPUT) found that rooibos "provided protection against oxidative stress of heart disease".

Herbal Teas for Colds and Useful Tips

A variety of teas can help if you have a mild cold. Put the herbal tea in a cup and add boiled water. Keep the cup covered for about 10 minutes, add honey when cool, and add lemon juice in order to preserve vitamins and nutrients.

Chamomile Tea

Chamomile tea has long been used as a traditional folk remedy for a wide range of health issues. Dried chamomile tea flowers are used to make the tea. This tea is most commonly known for its calming effects and frequently used as a sleep and relaxation aid, treating diabetes, lowering blood sugar, slowing or preventing osteoporosis, reducing inflammation, cancer treatment and prevention, treating cold symptoms, and for stomach problems. Infants and very young children should avoid chamomile tea, as well as those with severe allergies to pollen.

Peppermint Tea

Peppermint tea is sometimes referred as "the stomach healer" because it is known to soothe many stomach ailments, including stomach aches, stomach pain, stomach cramps, heartburn, gas/flatulence, indigestion and diarrhea. It also reduces fever, boosts immunity, treats respiratory disorders, prevents nausea and vomiting, protects heart health, reduces fever, removes bad breath, and helps with weight loss.

Lemon, Honey, and Ginger Tea

These tea ingredients have healing properties, facilitate cold symptoms, and enhance immunity. Lemon is rich in vitamin C, which fights against viruses and suppresses inflammation. Ginger is used to fight against digestive disorders. It stimulates the body's cleansing and inhibits inflammatory reactions. Honey suppresses coughing and promotes the growth of white blood cells, thus making the body more effective in fighting infections. **Method of preparation:** Add 2-3 pieces of thinly sliced ginger in a cup of boiling water and cover the cup. Wait about 5 minutes and add a teaspoon of honey and 1 teaspoon of freshly squeezed lemon juice. If you want more sweetness after tasting, add more honey.

Mint, Ginger, Garlic, Lemon, Honey, and Cayenne Pepper Tea

Mint tea helps to overcome the symptoms of flu and cold. The taste of this tea is unusual but effective. All these tea ingredients have healing properties in the fight against colds.
Method of preparation: Add 3-4 thinly sliced ginger pieces and 2-3 cloves of thinly sliced garlic. Add a pinch of cayenne pepper (they are very spicy) and a few leaves of dried or fresh mint. Pour hot boiled water and cover the cup, wait 5 minutes, squeeze 2-3 teaspoons of fresh lemon juice and add 1 teaspoon of honey.

Thyme (thymus vulgaris), Raspberry (rubus idaeus), Lemon, and Honey Tea

This tea can help fight against colds and flu.
Method of preparation: Put one dried raspberry stalk or their leaves and a teaspoon of dried thyme into a cup with boiling water, cover the cup, wait for 5 minutes. Add a slice of lemon and sweeten with a teaspoon of honey. Recommended to drink at bedtime, it promotes sweating and reduces fever.

Indian Tea

Indian tea warms up the body, allowing faster recovery.
Method of preparation: Add 2 teaspoons of black tea, ½ teaspoon of grated ginger, ½ teaspoon of cardamom, and 4 cloves to a large cup. Pour boiling water. Allow to stand for about 5 minutes, add honey and a little milk.

Ayurvedic Tea

This tea has been used since ancient times in holistic healthcare to achieve optimal health, energy and balance in life. Depending on a mix of botanicals, drinking an Ayurvedic blend can help enhance energy, promote emotional well-being, aid digestion, cleanse the body, calm nerves, and help to overcome coughing, and sneezing.
According to the National Institutes of Health, Ayurvedic is considered to be a form of complementary and alternative medicine. Dr. Suhas Kshirsagar's book called "The Hot Belly Diet" tells how to reset your metabolism and restore your body's natural balance to heal itself by drinking Ayurvedic tea. It consists of a blend of green tea, fennel seeds, coriander seeds, cumin seeds, fresh ginger, lemon juice. Some recipes add fresh turmeric root or turmeric powder. If you are going caffeine-free, you can use an herbal tea (like chamomile, mint, tulsi, or ginger) instead of green tea, or use white or black teas and other whole spices (like a cinnamon stick, whole clove, cardamom). Just mix it up a bit to your taste.

Ingredients:
4 cups water,
½ tablespoon thinly sliced ginger,
1 tablespoon thinly sliced fresh turmeric, or (½ -1 teaspoon ground powder),
1-2 teaspoons coriander seeds,
1-2 teaspoons cumin seeds,
1-2 teaspoons fennel seeds,
1-2 bags (tablespoons) green tea,
squeeze of lemon juice.

Preparation: To make the tea, place all seeds and roots in a French press and pour boiling water over the top. Let seep 5-10 minutes before plunging. Refill the French press as much as you like that day, simply reusing the same tea bag, seeds, roots. Alternatively, simmer all ingredients together for 5-10 minutes in a large pot and strain before drinking.

Spicy Green Tea

A great tool to help you overcome colds faster. Cayenne pepper and ginger improve blood circulation and promote sweating. Honey reduces throat pain while green tea contains many antioxidants and suppresses inflammatory processes.

Method of preparation: Mix 2 teaspoons of green tea with a pinch of cayenne pepper and 2 tablespoons of grated ginger. Cover the cup, hold for about 10 minutes, filter, and add 1 teaspoon of honey.

Turmeric Tea

Turmeric tea, high with antioxidants, helps prevent Alzheimer's disease and cancer, maintains ulcerative colitis remission, boosts the immune system, lowers cholesterol, reduces arthritis symptoms, helps cardiovascular health, longevity, and managing diabetes. It's also good for mental health and weight loss.

Method of preparation: Boil 3-4 cups of water, add 2 teaspoons of turmeric, simmer for about 5-10 minutes, strain the tea into another container. Add honey, milk, and fresh squeezed lemon or orange juice to taste.

Spicy Antibacterial Tea

Extremely spicy tea which can help to overcome the first symptoms of cold.

Method of preparation: Add 1 clove of chopped garlic, 1 teaspoon grated ginger, a pinch of cayenne pepper, ½ teaspoon of turmeric, and a pinch of black pepper to a cup. Put the boiling water in the cup, cover it for 10 minutes, squeeze in half of a fresh lemon, and add 1 teaspoon of honey.

Rosehip Tea

Rosehip Tea is not only suitable for drinking when one has a cold, but also as a daily tea drinking ritual as the sloes are rich in vitamin C.

Method of preparation: Add 3 tablespoons of crushed and dried sloes to ½ liter of boiling water. Filter and pour in a thermos. Drink half a glass 4 times a day.

Tea with Jam.

This long-forgotten and rare tea is made with boiled berries (jam) or fresh cranberry berries mashed with sugar. The tea will warm your insides with its pleasant aroma and taste. If you have the flu, this raspberry, blueberry, cherry, or cranberry tea will help and strengthen the immune system.

Method of preparation: Add 1-2 teaspoons of boiled berries (raspberries, cherries, blueberries, cranberries or other berries) to hot water and stir.

The best way to prepare jams from berries is to pick them from your own garden or from local farmers, though one can use those you've bought in a store.

To prevent colds and strengthen your immunity, stay in the fresh air as much as possible, and even try to go out in cold weather. Make sure you consume enough vitamin C. Vitamin C is abundant in fruits such as lemons, oranges, kiwi fruit, and berries. Also, it is important to eat lots of different vegetables. It's better to breathe through the nose than through the mouth. In the morning, choose a contrast shower, exercise, and try to travel short distances on foot. Adjust your diet by choosing healthy and nutritious foods. All this can help prevent colds. The aforementioned tea recipes can help you get better sooner.

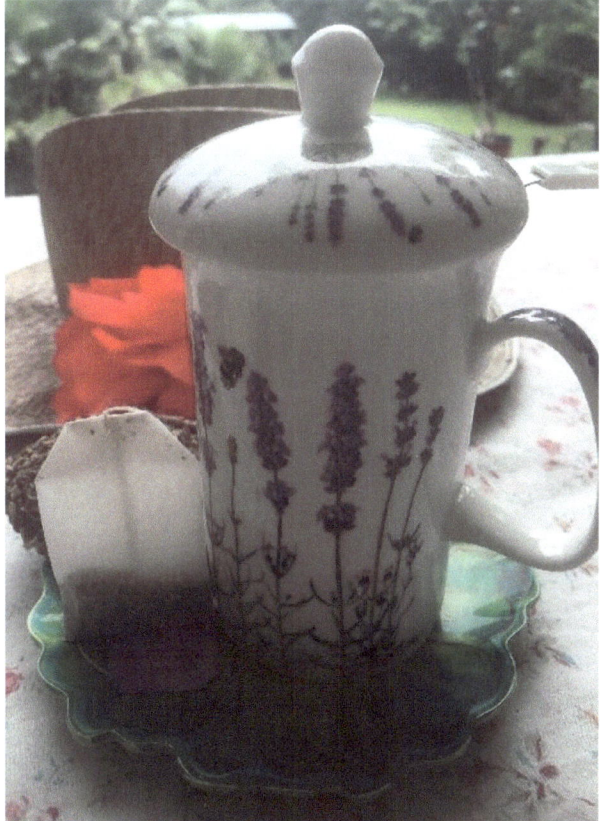

Apple Cider Vinegar

It is said that Hippocrates treated his patients with vinegar 400 years ago. Although the benefits of vinegar have been forgotten in the 20th century, experts say that vinegar can be an excellent elixir of beauty and health. The beneficial properties of this product are mentioned in the Bible, as well as in ancient Roman, Greek, and Egyptian writings. In the middle ages, doctors disinfected their hands with apple vinegar during the raging plague. Apple cider vinegar contains vitamins, amino acids, fiber, pectin, and microelements.

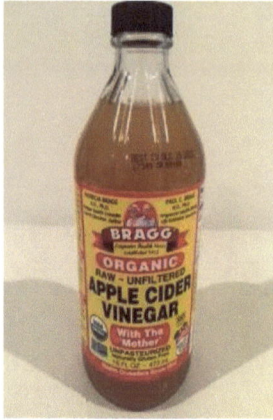

Apple cider vinegar has an antibacterial, antifungal effect. Therefore, it destroys harmful bacteria and fungi and helps to restore intestinal microflora, reduce inflammation, and treat fungus. If you want to use vinegar at home, use only organic, unfiltered, and unpasteurized apple vinegar. Consult your dermatologist and family physician before usage.

Intestine. Apple cider vinegar improves digestion and stimulates gastric juice release. It is saturated with amino acids and vitamins that have inflammatory properties and it can protect the intestines from infections, eliminate harmful bacteria, and help maintain healthy intestinal flora. While using apple cider vinegar, intestinal peristalsis is improved. It is recommended to drink a glass of boiled water with 1 teaspoon of vinegar and 1 teaspoon of honey before a meal.

Osteoporosis. Symptoms of the disease are that the bones become thin and brittle. As the bones become more fragile, they can break. You can mitigate the course of the disease by natural means. Grind 10 eggshells with a coffee grinder and add enough apple cider vinegar to cover the shells. Leave in a dark place for a week. Take one half of a teaspoon before bedtime for one month.

Insect Bites. Apply apple cider vinegar to the bite site, wait until dry, and apply again. This will reduce the itching on the bite site.

Hair Rinsing. Rinse your hair with apple cider vinegar after washing. The hair will be brighter and more vivacious. Mix water and cider in equal parts, and rinse twice a week. If hair loss starts, rub the scalp with the water and vinegar mixture. Do this before head washing.

Overweight. Apple cider vinegar helps to reduce appetite. Therefore, it helps to regulate weight and accelerates metabolic processes. To lose weight, it is recommended to drink a glass of warm water with one teaspoon of apple vinegar cider 3-4 times a day before meals. After a couple of months, you may notice a significantly reduced body weight. It is suggested that vinegar burns fat, and that pectin found in vinegar removes cholesterol from the body.

Sore throat. Mix 1 tablespoon of apple cider vinegar, 2 tablespoons of water, 1 tablespoon of honey, ¼ teaspoon of cayenne pepper. Take small sips and swallow slowly so that your throat will come in contact with this tea. This tea should be sipped every few hours. This recipe is recommended by medical nurse Bonnie K. McMillen of Pittsburgh University.

Salad with Apple Cider Vinegar. Add broccoli, asparagus, or salad leaves, and mix the following ingredients: 1 tablespoon of apple cider vinegar, 1 tablespoon of squeezed lime juice (or lemon), ½ tablespoon of chopped garlic, a pinch of pepper, and freshly crushed basil leaves.

Recovering forces. Apple cider vinegar is suitable for use with honey because it regulates the balance of herbs and alkalis in the body. This product helps a person to recover quickly from illness and stress and gives energy. In the morning, it is advisable to drink one glass of boiled warm water with 1 teaspoon of apple cider vinegar and 1 teaspoon of honey.

Diabetes. Arizona State University invited two groups of 11 volunteers who had Grade 2 diabetes to participate in a study. For both groups, the researchers used the prescribed medications typically administered by a doctor. In one group, each volunteer drank 2 tablespoons of vinegar with one ounce of cheese before going to bed. The other 11 volunteers had to drink 2 tablespoons of water with the cheese. In the morning, the volunteers who had used the vinegar had a lower sugar content than those who had used the water.

Facial toner. Apple cider vinegar (ACV) is a perfect toner for the face. Mix it with tea or an herbal tea infusion and drink. Soon after, the face will be cleaner, more beautiful, and more elastic. This lotion could be applied to all types of skin, says Dr. Karen Hammerman, a cosmetic dermatologist at Vanguard Dermatology in New York City. I dilute one tablespoon of ACV with a few drops of water and apply with a cotton ball three to four times a week. If you have extremely sensitive skin, try adding more water to the mixture and use less frequently.

Clean up make-up brushes. Dr. Karen Hammerman suggests combining one cup of warm water with one teaspoon of ACV, and one or two thick slices of lemon to scent the concoction. Clean the brushes with the mixture, rinse with water, and lay out to dry.

Apple cider vinegar should not be used by those with urinal acid-based circulatory problems, stomach or small intestine stomach ulcers, gastritis, chronic and acute hepatitis, and kidney and urinary tract stone disease. Vinegar, like any acid, can also damage the tooth enamel and the stomach mucous membrane, especially when taken on an empty stomach. Increasing the amount of vinegar can seriously damage your health. Caution should be taken by people who are sensitive to mold because vinegar and its preserved foods can cause allergic reactions.

Chapter 12

EAT CLEAN, GET LEAN

Health is not about the weight you lose, but about the life you gain!
– Dr. Josh Axe

The Eat Clean Rules

There are six simple strategies for a smarter diet:

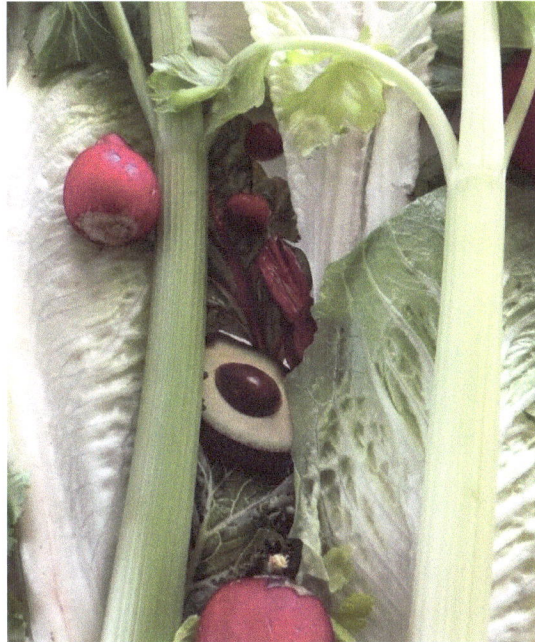

1. **Get Back to Basics.** The primary tenet of clean eating is to eat more food in its natural state, such as unsalted nuts, grass-fed and free-range meats, and whole fruits and vegetables. It is common sense, really, but the truth is that much of what we consume today is chemically altered, such as "the maltodextrins and high-fructose corn syrups and the stuff that doesn't exist outside of a factory", as stated by Tamara Duker Freuman, a clinical dietitian based in New York. Try to allow yourself two more servings a day of real food and you'll be on your way to better health.

2. **Think Outside the Box.** Most food that comes in a box is processed in some way, which means it could either contain additives that you don't need or that some of the food's essential goodness has been stripped away. Therefore, it is worth choosing foods with the least amount of processing. For example, you're much better off eating a fig than a Fig Newton. The closer a food is to its original form, the better it is for you.

3. **Check the Label.** "Read the ingredients list," says dietician Laura Georgy. The healthiest foods are the ones that contain the fewest ingredients. As Michelle Dudash, author of Clean Eating for Busy Families, states, "If you can't pronounce an ingredient, you probably shouldn't eat it."

4. **Know the Enemy.** Certain ingredients have no place in your pantry at all because they have been shown to affect cholesterol, blood pressure, or blood sugar. These five should never cross your lips.

- **Trans-fats**: look for "partially hydrogenated vegetable oil," "hydrogenated vegetable oil," and "shortening" in cookies, crackers, and microwave popcorn. The by-product of hydrogenation, trans-fat, raises bad (LDL) cholesterol and lowers good (HDL) cholesterol, thereby increasing the risk of heart attack and stroke.
- **Food coloring:** Take out your reading glasses and look for "blue1," "blue 2," "citrus red 2," "green 2," "orange B," "red 40," "yellow 5," and "yellow 6" in baked goods, cereals, and condiments. Synthetic food dyes have been linked with tumors in animal studies.
- **Artificial sweeteners**: Watch out for "acesulfame-K," "saccharin," and "aspartame" on a food that claims to be "low sugar" or "low carb."
- **High-fructose corn syrup:** Look for "high-fructose corn syrup" and "corn sweetener" in everything from bread to salad dressings. These concentrated simple sugars cause a cascade of blood sugar and insulin spikes and drops that may have the unintended consequence of making us crave even more high-sugar, high-fat food, no matter how much we've just eaten.
- **Nitrates and nitrites:** Scan smoked meat and jerky for the deceptively healthy-sounding ingredient "celery juice." These are undercover additives used to preserve the red color of the meat and are associated with ovarian and kidney cancers, according to the long-running NIH-AARP Diet and Health Study.

5. **Shop Smarter**: The following foods offer major health benefits as they are low in sugar and salt and high in fiber and savory flavors.

- **Hummus:** The protein in hummus keeps you fuller for longer and its high iron content increases energy.
- **Peppercorns**: Piperine, the substance that gives black pepper its pungency, blocks the formation of fat cells.
- **Tuna and salmon pouches**: Cold-water fish support the neurological function, are anti-inflammatory, and for those with cardiac issues, eating tuna and salmon has a mild blood-thinning effect.
- **Gelatin**: Rich in amino acids, particularly glycine, which supports skin, hair, joint, nail, and gut health.
- **Sprouted-grain bread**: This chewy bread can provide more vitamin C and other nutrients than loaves made with flour. Always choose whole-grain bread over white.
- **Garlic powder:** Nearly as beneficial as fresh garlic, the powdered form strengthens the immune system, reduces cholesterol, and fights cancer.
- **Chia seeds:** Add these super seeds to smoothies and salads for a dose of healthy fats, fiber, and protein.

- **Oats:** They contain bone-beneficial iron and magnesium, plus fiber, which is a prebiotic-food that feeds the good bacteria in your gut. As supported by Food Guru Michael Pollan, "I soak my oatmeal with water and sometimes a little yogurt so it begins to ferment; this makes it more nutritious and easier to digest."
- **Fermented foods:** Miso, sauerkraut, and kimchi with live active cultures are full of probiotics, all of which aid digestion.
- **Quinoa and whole grain pasta:** These can provide the basis for fast, fiber-rich meals on those evenings when you find you don't have much time to cook.
- **Seasonal fruits and vegetables:** Asparagus, green beans, and cruciferous vegetables such as broccoli and cauliflower contain sulfur compounds that help you eliminate the toxins that cause oxidative damage—the precursor to most diseases. Blue and purple berries contain resveratrol, which promotes healthy aging by reducing inflammation and blood sugar, in addition to supporting the cardiovascular system.
- **Lean meat:** Buy chicken or lean beef rather than fattier alternatives. If possible, choose grass-fed or sustainably raised options.

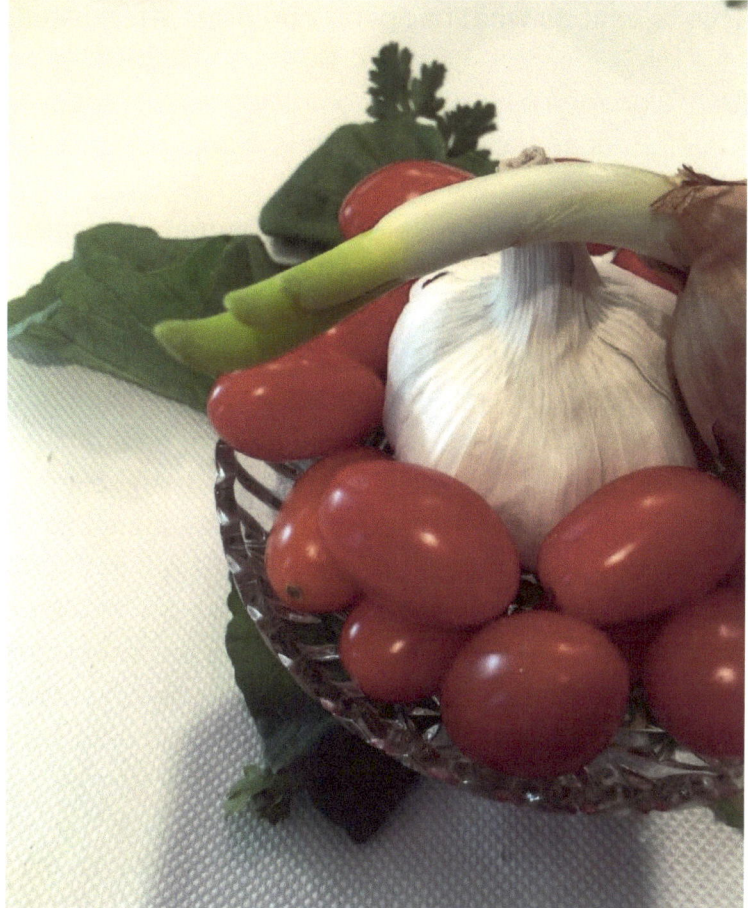

6. **Eat at home.** Conversely, people who prepare most of their own meals at home eat less, even when they then do choose to eat out.

This is exactly what happens one hour after drinking a can of Coke

"Just stop for a second and do nothing. Pay attention to what your mind is telling you".
— Jeff Bridges. Actor, singer, and producer

An infographic by The Renegade Pharmacist breaks down exactly what happens while you are drinking a can of Coke. It vividly describes every bodily response that occurs from the first sip, right through to 60 minutes after drinking the entire can.

1. During the first 10 minutes, 8-10 teaspoons of sugar—the contents of the can—enters the body, which is the entire recommended daily sugar intake.
2. After 20 minutes, the sugar content of the jump causes an insulin burst. Your liver responds to this and converts the sugars into fat.
3. After 40 minutes, the caffeine present in the "Coca-Cola" is absorbed. There is a sudden rise in blood pressure, which the liver responds to, putting sugar into the bloodstream. Certain brain receptors are stimulated, which reduces drowsiness.
4. After 45 minutes, the body stimulates the production of dopamine and stimulates the pleasure centers in the brain. The drug heroin also works in this way.
5. After 60 minutes, phosphoric acid is bound to the calcium, magnesium, and zinc in your lower intestine, which provides additional stimulus to the metabolism. A large dose of sugar and sweeteners stimulates the release of calcium in the urine.
6. After 60 minutes, the urine released from the body includes all the calcium, magnesium, and zinc trace elements that are beneficial to your bones. Also, the body is deprived of water, sodium, and electrolytes.

The key information to take away from this is that as you consume soda and it goes through your body, essential vitamins and minerals are expelled from your body. Aside from the effects that soda causes internally, dark carbonated drinks also increase the likelihood of staining your teeth. While having just one can give you that momentary "boost" you need, the amount of sugar a soda can contains is also well over your recommended daily intake.

So, the next time you're thinking about grabbing a cold soda, just remember that in the amount of time it takes you to finish the can, you're causing a lot more long-term damage than you think.

An interesting story: It was in 1886, just 21 years after the American Civil War. At that time, in Atlanta, Georgia, pharmacist John Pemberton was working in his garden. The French Coca-Cola — "an excellent tonic medicine that helps regain strength and energy" — had already been invented, as well as a lemon and orange elixir.

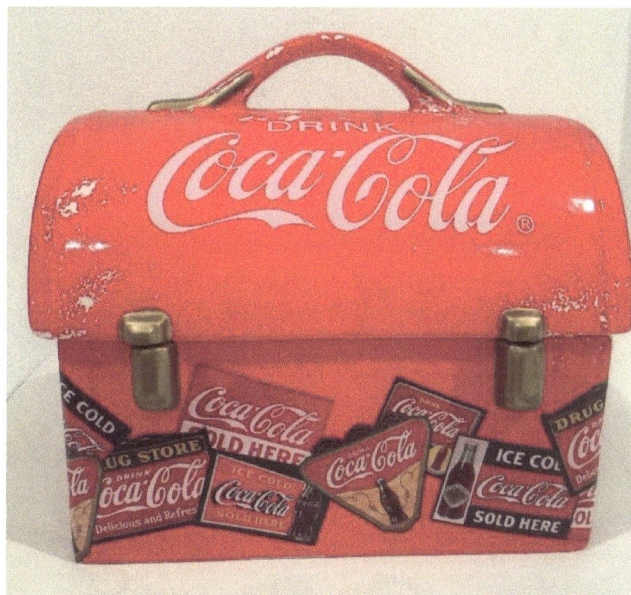

In his garden, John cooked a potion in a copper pot over an open fire, and with that, he created a new drug to combat nervous breakdowns and headaches. When he was satisfied with the recipe, he took it to the Jacob pharmacy, telling one of the assistants that it was syrup mixed with water and cooled with ice. Having tasted the liquid, they both agreed that it was delicious. However, a different assistant accidentally poured a glass of sparkling water into the potion. Then, with this unexpected discovery, the two men decided not to sell it as a means of a headache reliever but rather as a soft drink; specifically, a lemonade and ginger beer substitute. The drink was then called Coke, because it used coca leaves and kola nuts in its production. Kola nuts are fruits from the kola tree, a genus (cola).

In 1886, according to the Coca-Cola Company, Pemberton sold his 25 gallons of syrup. He received $50, but had spent $73.96 on advertising.

Five years later, druggist Asa Candler purchased the rights to the drink and began to promote it across the country, making it available in all states and territories by 1895. He sold the rights to bottle the product in 1899 and the first bottling plant was opened in Chattanooga, followed by one in Atlanta.

Available in 155 countries, 393 million bottles of Coca-Cola are consumed on a daily basis. Now, Pemberton is not recognized for inventing a drug to treat headaches or nervous breakdowns, but he is known for having invented one of the world's favorite beverages.

(Text prepared according to the book "Successful Error")

What's Worse Than Sugar?

"If you do not care for your body, where are you going to live?"
— Unknown

1. **High-fructose corn syrup**. Food manufacturers began substituting high-fructose corn syrup for sugar in the 1970s, however, its use skyrocketed in the 1990s when people turned to low-fat foods and forgot about calories and sugar content. Experts warn that high-fructose corn syrup is making us fat.

   Dietary experts and scientists are singling out high-fructose corn syrup as a reason for the startling rise in obesity in America and a related increase in diabetes cases. Storey and other health experts point out that a lack of exercise, not just calories, contributes to obesity.

2. **Acesulfame-potassium**. Acesulfame-potassium is 200 times sweeter than sugar. Discovered in 1967 and approved by the FDA in 1988, the FDA says studies show no carcinogenic effects, but critics say there hasn't been enough research. The Center for Science in the Public Interest (CSPI), a consumer advocate for nutrition and health, cited the possible cancer and thyroid risks of this sweetener.

3. **Aspartame**. Aspartame is 180-220 times sweeter than sugar. Discovered in 1965 and approved by the FDA in 1981, some researchers have raised concerns about its links to brain cancer, leukemia, and lymphomas, but the FDA and international food safety commissions say reviews of the many studies and clinical trials on aspartame show that it bears no links to cancer. CSPI recommends avoiding aspartame, citing possible health risks.

4. **Saccharin**. Saccharin is 200 times sweeter than sugar. Discovered in 1879 and approved by the FDA in 1958, a number of studies have linked saccharin to bladder cancer in rats, leading the FDA to recommend a ban in 1977. Instead, congress required all products containing saccharin to carry a warning label. However, human studies have shown no consistent cancer links. Therefore, in the year 2000, saccharin was delisted as a carcinogen and the warning label requirement was repealed. CSPI says to avoid saccharin.

5. **Sucralose.** Sucralose is 600 times sweeter than sugar. Discovered in 1976 and approved by the FDA in 1998, sucralose is made with real sugar and chlorine. Studies have found no links to cancer, according to the FDA, and the CSPI says it

appears to be safe, but warns of health risks if frequently used in conjunction with acesulfame- potassium.

6. **Neotame.** It is 7,000 to 13,000 times sweeter than sugar. Discovered in 1965 and approved by the FDA in 2002, the FDA says there are no adverse effects when ingested at levels used in foods. The CSPI says it appears to be safe.

7. **Stevia.** Stevia is 300 times sweeter than sugar. First discovered by a group of French researchers, who isolated the plant's sweetness in 1931, Stevia had previously been used for centuries in Central and South America. FDA approved in December 2008, this calorie-free natural sweetener has been used in Japan for decades and elsewhere in Asia and Latin America. Rat studies have shown reduced sperm count, infertility, smaller offspring, and DNA mutation. CSPI urges caution, warning that stevia needs to be tested further.

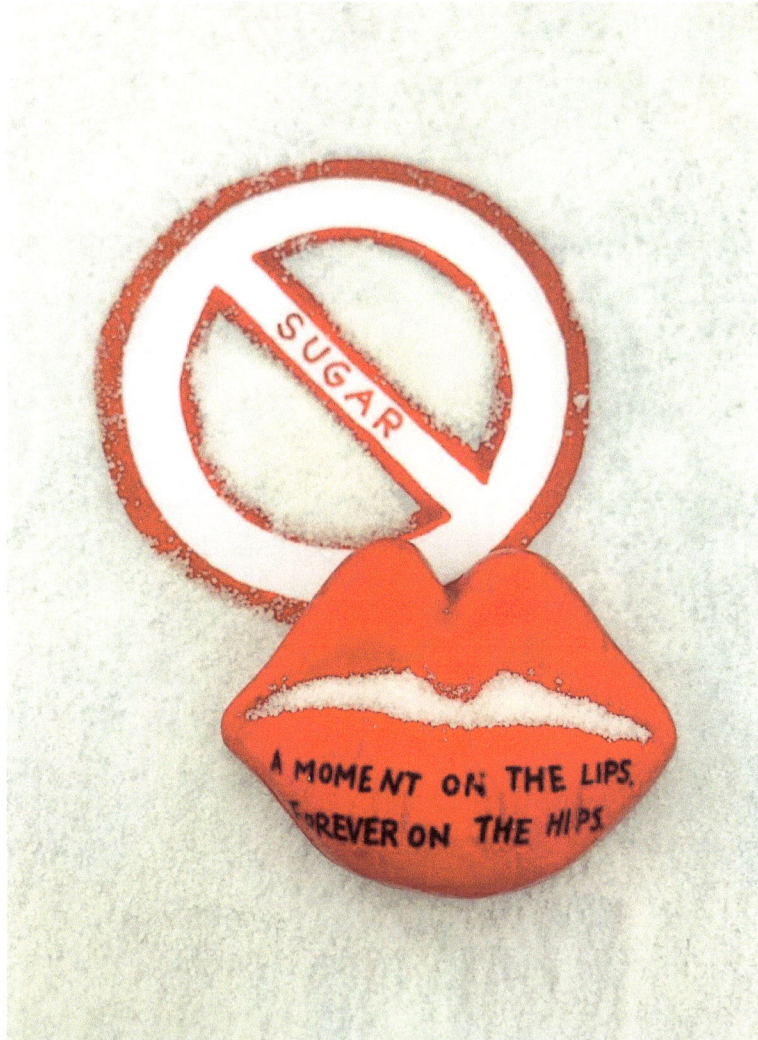

Chapter 13

OILS

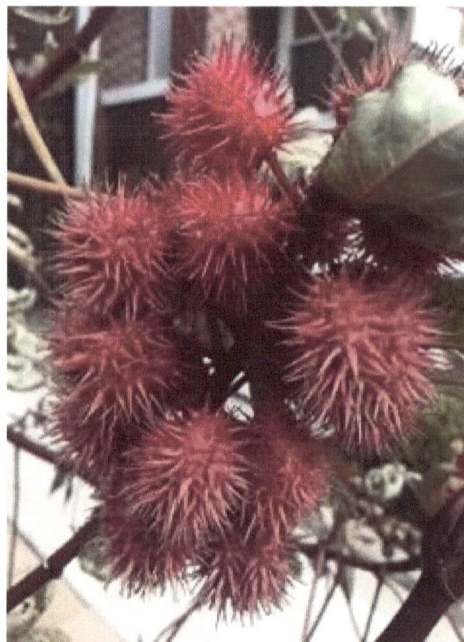

Ricinus Tree

"The Secret of Happiness lies in looking at all the wonders of the world and never forgetting the two drops of oil in the spoon."
(Proverb)

Coconut Oil

The coconut *(Cocos nucifera)* is a palm tree of the Arecaceae family. The coconut seed, or fruit, botanically, is not a nut, but technically a drupe. The word "coco," meaning "head," comes from the tree indentations on the coconut shell that resemble facial features. For centuries the coconut oil tree has been called "the tree of life." Virtually every part of it can be used or consumed. In Sanskrit it is called kalpavriksha or "tree of heaven." Organic coconut oil is called pressed and never chemically treated during production. It is extracted from the kernel of mature coconut. Coconut Oil is an excellent and natural remedy for skin and hair care without any harmful side effects.

Hair Care

Coconut oil is one of the best natural remedies for the hair. It helps to maintain a healthy hair structure, stimulates growth, and gives a high-quality shine for your hair, in addition to helping prevent hair loss. It is also an effective remedy for protein deficiency, which can result in a loss of hair or make the hair look unhealthy. Coconut oil works well as a conditioner and helps to repair damaged hair if you use the coconut oil daily after bathing or a shower. It contains the essential proteins needed to feed and heal damaged hair. Regular massage of the head with coconut oil will ensure that no dandruff occurs, even if your scalp is very dry. The oil is easily absorbed into the hair and will not leave an unpleasant feeling of greasiness. It will also help to protect the hair and scalp from lice and their eggs.

How to use
The simplest and most popular way to use coconut oil is simply to rub it into your hair and hair ends, which will protect the hair ends from splitting; if you have very oily hair, do not rub the roots, just the hair surface. Massage your head with oil for about 3 minutes to

improve circulation in the scalp. The oil is kept on for 1 hour, but the best results will be achieved if you leave coconut oil overnight with a shower cap or wrap the hair with a cloth and sleep (put a towel on the pillow in order not to make it greasy). In the morning, wash your hair with shampoo or 100% black soap. Allow your hair to dry completely and rub a small amount of oil directly into the hair. You will feel the difference immediately.

Hair Spray. Ingredients:

- 1 cup of water,
- 1 long leaf of aloe vera,
- 1 tablespoon coconut oil,
- Juice from one onion.

Preparation: In a small pot, boil 1 cup of water. Add small pieces of aloe vera and boil for 5 minutes. Drain the liquid, add 1 tablespoon of coconut oil. Mix well. Pour liquid in a 12 oz. (375 ml) spray bottle. Add onion juice and shake it well. Spray on hair roots, leaving for 40 minutes. Rinse afterwards. Repeat twice a week. After 14 days your hair will look stronger, thicker, and reduce hair loss.

Coconut Oil for Skin

This oil will serve as a perfect massage oil and moisturizer for all types of skin, particularly protecting dry and scaly skin. This oil protects against wrinkles and slows down the skin aging processes. It also helps to treat psoriasis, dermatitis, eczema, and some skin-causing infections.

Other Uses for Coconut Oil

1. Make-up Remover. Apply on a cotton swab and gently scrub the face.

2. Face scrub. Add some soda to the coconut oil and gently scrub the skin of the face. After washing it, any residue will be absorbed after a few minutes.

3. Eye Cream. The oil moisturizes and softens the skin around the eyes, minimizing wrinkles.

4. Facial cleanser. Gently massage the face and neck with coconut oil, then wash well. If you wash daily, the skin will become smoother and cleaner.

5. Moisturizer. Coconut oil can accelerate wound healing, improve skin hydration, and prevent moisture loss. Use coconut oil as a lotion to liven up the skin and make it more beautiful. Coconut oil is suitable for cracked heels and elbows, where it softens and nourishes the skin.

6. Body scrub. Make a mixture of coconut oil and brown sugar. Coconut oil has antifungal properties, so it is perfectly suitable for a foot scrub. You can also make a body scrub by mixing coconut oil with coffee.

7. Leg and armpit depilation. The commercial depilatory creams are filled with chemicals and are expensive—use coconut oil instead. It is a natural remedy with an antibacterial effect and a wonderful aroma.

8. Moisten dry hands. Coconut oil it is a great tool for maintaining your hands. Rub your hands with coconut oil and give it some time to absorb.

9. Facial mask. Mix a teaspoon of coconut oil with one teaspoon of sour cream and ¾ banana. Apply this mashed mass on the face and neck, hold for 20 minutes. Rinse with warm water.

10. Shaving Cream. If you have sensitive skin or if you are sensitive to the chemicals found in the shaving creams, try coconut oil instead.

Unlike other oils, coconut oil is solid. Its melting point is 24-25ºC, above 75 degrees of F. In order to use it, in most cases the oil will need to be heated. This can be done by leaving it in the sun or placing in warm water. It does not need to be stored in the refrigerator.

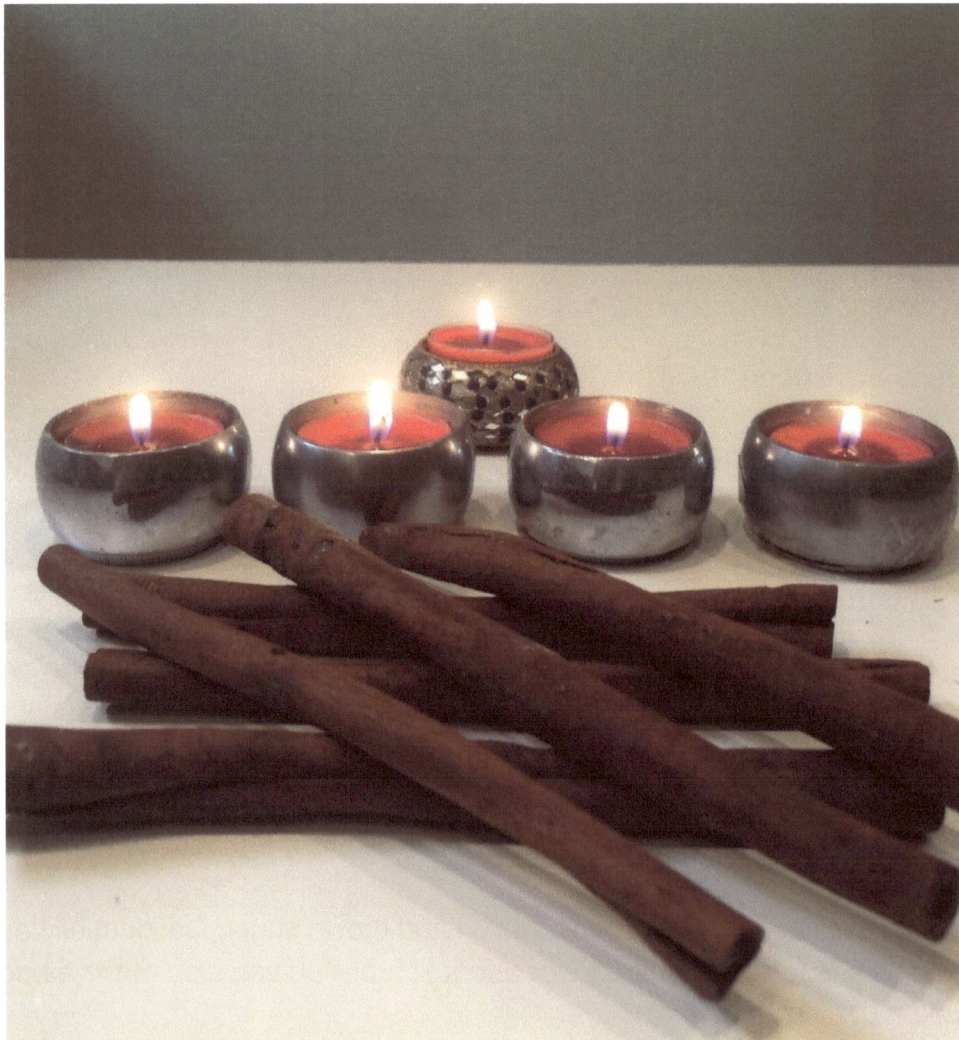

Castor Oil

Castor Oil is extracted from the ricinus tree (Ricinus communis) seeds, from the family Euphorbiaceae. The castor oil plant is native to the Ethiopian region of East Africa. The beans are oblong and light brown mottled with dark brown spots. The seeds are only toxic if the outer shell is broken or chewed. Ricin is contained in the bean pulp following the separation of the oil from the bean. The plant has very large, beautiful leaves that resemble a chestnut. The fruits of the plant are small box-like fruits, which contain three beautiful large seeds that shine like marble. The seeds have a non-drying oil distinguished for its special properties and widely known in various industries. Castor oil is a safe product that has been used as a medicine since the times of the ancient Egyptians, who commonly used it as an internal and external medicine. The Egyptians put compresses with castor oil on open wounds and sometimes did not remove the compress for a week or two. They also combined honey with castor. Honey was used as an antiseptic for the treatment of burns.

Doctor Robin Murphy was interested in castor oil therapy and made some studies, thereby accumulating a wealth of medical knowledge about castor oil and its use in practice.

Usage of Castor Oil

The ricinus tree is called the Palma Christi because sometimes this plant treats only by touch. In Egypt, this castor oil was called digim, which is a thick and viscous oil. It is an excellent oil not only for hair and scalp, but also for eyelashes and ankles. The oil has antifungal, antiviral, and antibacterial properties, therefore, it is an effective remedy for the treatment of head-related infections, particularly fungi. In medicine, castor oil is used as a laxative for intestinal cleansing. If you drink one or two tablespoons of castor oil, laxative effects begin after five to six hours. This oil is used to empty the intestine before a radiological or instrumental intestinal examination or colon surgery.

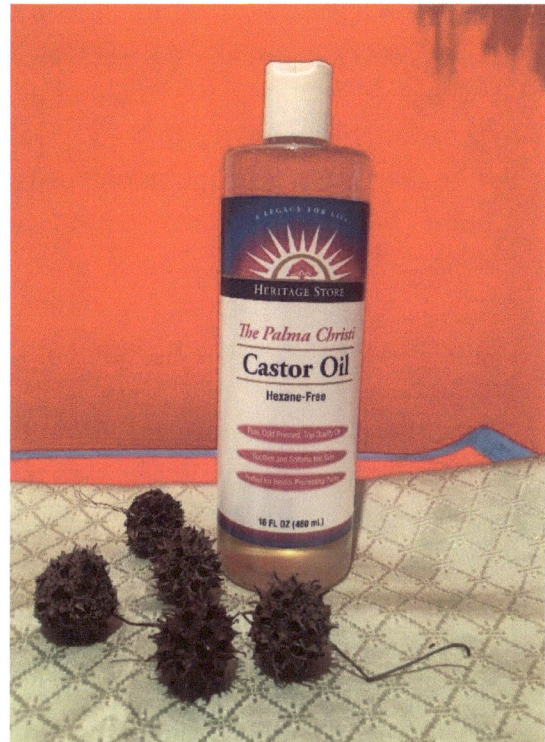

Hair Care

Castor Oil has been used to cherish the health and beauty of hair for many years. It has antibacterial and antifungal effects. Castor oil contains important nutrients, vitamin E, minerals, and Omega 6 and Omega 9 fats. This is a classic beauty remedy that helps to regrow long hair and eyelashes.

It is believed that the regular use of castor oil can accelerate hair growth from 2 to 5 times, creating hair that is thicker, looser, and shinier. Castor oil is rubbed into the scalp to stop hair loss and scaling. Castor acid, which is found in castor oil, improves the blood circulation of the scalp and promotes hair growth, helping to restore the natural moisture of the scalp and protecting against the harmful chemicals that occur in some hair care products.

Leave the castor oil in your hair and put on a shower cap or wrap your hair with a cloth for 3 hours or overnight for best results. Oil is well absorbed at night and it will be easier to wash your hair in the morning. To make it easier to wash your hair after castor oil, you can rub it with a conditioner before washing.

Arthritis. Castor oil has been known as a natural remedy for arthritis since ancient times. It reduces inflammation and aching muscles; therefore, it can be used as massage oil. Castor oil is like a balsam for the joints, anesthetizing and lubricating them. Massage your knees and feet every morning and evening and for five minutes until the oil is well absorbed into the skin. To increase the effect, the rubbed spots may also be warmed. Heat dilates the blood vessels and oil absorbs better. (Heat the oil, moisten it with a flannel cloth, and cover the desired area of the body, covering this cloth with a towel). Castor oil softens the skin and acts as a joint ointment. Over time, all joints calcify and harden. Greased and absorbed oil lubricates the joints, helping them to regenerate and renew their flexibility. Dr. Robin Murphy suggests applying a lot of castor oil several times a day in cases of arthritis. People whose necks are sore from sitting in front of the TV or at the computer will benefit from neck massage with castor oil. Due to the thickness and viscosity of castor oil, it needs to be rubbed into the joints well because only well-absorbed oil heals. Regular rubbing of oil in the joints is a common way to treat people who cannot move their hands or feet and those who use a wheelchair.

Spondylitis is a condition where the spinal bones grow together, while rheumatism is the rigidity or paralysis of the joints. Many people find relief after two months of working with castor oil.

Colds, flu, headaches. In these cases, the forehead, neck, and sinus nodules are rubbed with castor oil. Rub the chest with oil if you have a cold or are coughing. The Egyptians used to rub the belly-button also. Doctor Robin Murphy does this every day in the shower. Some mothers find rubbing castor or olive oils on their baby's belly will help with colic.

Warts, calluses, and foot sores. Rubbing your feet with castor oil softens the skin, helping moles, calluses, and warts to disappear. Use large quantities of oil and massage for five minutes.

Skin and muscle. Rubbing castor oil on split skin on elbows, knees, and scaly skin is beneficial in combating psoriasis. You could treat varicose veins with castor oil compresses, changing the bandages several times a day. The oil has a good effect in muscular atrophy and multiple sclerosis.

Improve facial skin. Apply castor oil on the face in the evening, making sure to gently wipe away any excess with gauze after 20 minutes. The best way to use castor oil is to rub a small amount into the skin. Leave for 2-3 hours and wash. Do this in a cooler climate, such as in winter, because it can cause discomfort in warmer weather. By doing this daily for several months you will renew your skin, tighten it, and eliminate acne scars and small wrinkles.

Foot heels. Use if they are rough and cracked. Start with warm salt and soda baths, clean the soaked skin, then rub it with castor oil and apply a wool or cotton swab with oil on the heels. After several procedures, the heels will heal and will become soft and resistant to cracking.

If new shoes rub on your toes, apply oil and the sore will quickly be treated. To soften the leather of shoes, rub them with castor oil. If you live in a village and your cow has warts on its teats, the perfect treatment is to rub them with castor oil. Also, castor oil can help with hemorrhoids.

Mix with Other Oils

1. As castor oil is viscous, it can be mixed with other oils. For example, mixing castor oil, olive oil, and rosemary in equal parts creates a hair oil that smells wonderful.
2. Add a tablespoon of lavender oil to castor oil and it will give a pleasant scent to your hair.
3. Mix 1 tablespoon of castor oil with 1 tablespoon of coconut oil. Divide the hair into 2 equal parts along the middle of the head. Mix well. Rub the mixture from the root of the hair to the hair ends with a soaked cotton swab or use a dropping pipette on the head until it is completely covered with a thin layer of mixture. Massage your head for 5 minutes. Wrap your hair with a warm cloth or put on a shower cap and leave on the hair for 2-3 hours or more. Rinse as usual.

This method will protect your hair from damage, increase growth, and nourish your hair and scalp.

The most important thing is to select 100% pure, unrefined, hexane-free, cold pressed oil.

Pregnant women and infants should **avoid** castor oil. There is evidence from animal studies and case reports that castor oil might be dangerous for the fetus if taken in early pregnancy due to the possible dehydration effects of induced diarrhea. However, when researches have looked at using castor oil at the end of pregnancy at term to induce labor, studies have found that it is effective at inducing labor although dehydration may weaken the birth and can cause overly-fierce contractions.

Treatments using plants and their oils require patience and persistence. The results are felt gradually, not immediately

Argan Oil

Argan Oil (Argania spinosa). Derived from seeds of the Moroccan argan tree of the Sapotaceae family, argan oil is also known as liquid gold. Rich in fatty acids and vitamin E, this oil is commonly used in cosmetics and for hair and skin care.

Argan Oil for Skin. Argan Oil does not leave an unpleasant feeling of greasiness after use. It easily absorbs into the skin, does not clog pores, and helps regulate the natural fatness of the skin. This oil can be used day and night as it is easily absorbed. Argan Oil suppresses skin aging, makes wrinkles less visible, and gives the skin a shine. Its antioxidants protect the skin from harmful environmental effects and free radicals. Pamper your face and neck with a few drops of argan oil before going to bed. Your lips will become elastic and soft, especially in cold or dry weather conditions.

Hair Conditioner. Argan Oil is beneficial for hair due to its high content of vitamin E. It promotes healthy hair growth, moisturizes dry scalp, helps brittle hair, reduces dandruff, and restores hair after chemical damage. Argan Oil, unlike other conditioners, does not need to be washed out after application. It easily absorbs into the hair and leaves no residues behind—you just need to choose the right amount. Rub a few drops of pure oil into your palms and comb your hair with your fingers followed by a gentle scalp massage. Do this on damp or gently towel-dried hair. This will help you to have a healthy scalp, promote hair growth, and prevent hair split ends.

Hair Loss. Wash your head before applying the oil and dry it with a cloth. The scalp must be clean and have open hair follicles. Rub your fingers with argan oil and massage your head in circular movements for 15 minutes. This will allow the oil to penetrate the hair follicles. Repeat this procedure 3 times a week, and once the hair loss stabilizes, do it once a week.

Hair Mask. Massage a large amount of the oil into your scalp at bedtime, wrap your head with a cloth or shower cap, and leave it overnight. Wash your hair in the morning as usual.

Macadamia Oil

Macadamia nut oil comes from Macadamia ternifolia, which is an Australian tree and part of the plant family Proteaceae. Macadamia nuts are grown in Australia, South Africa, and the Hawaiian Islands. This oil contains a lot of nutrients, such as minerals, vitamin B, and vitamin E, and contains the highest concentration of palmitoleic acid (omega 7) of all plants. This acid promotes skin self-regulating functions. Macadamia Oil is called magic due to its special health and beauty properties for the skin and hair. It is suitable for all types of skin, is easily absorbed into the skin and hair, and it does not leave an unpleasant feeling of greasy skin.

Hair care. This oil is very well absorbed into the scalp and it is especially suitable for treating dry hair. It stimulates hair growth, moisturizes hair, reduces the amount of dandruff, and gives the hair a beautiful shine. This oil is often used as a hair conditioner. Rub a wet head with a few drops of this oil and let it soak in for at least 15-30 minutes. Rinsing afterwards is optional.

Hair Mask. Pour ¼ cup of macadamia oil into a cup, add a few drops of tea tree oil or chamomile essential oil, and add some aloe vera gel. These products complement each other and stimulate hair growth, moisturize the scalp, cure dandruff, and make the hair shiny. Before applying the mask to your hair, wash your hair and dry it with a cloth. Take a little of the mask on your palm and rub your arms, then gently apply the rest of the mask to your hair. Rinse with warm water after 10 minutes. Do this procedure twice a week.

Macadamia Oil for Skin. Use macadamia oil after showering. Apply a small amount of oil to your entire body and face. It absorbs quickly and provides protection from aging.

Other Uses

1. Make-up Remover. Pour ¾ cup of oil into a glass, add 1 capsule of vitamin E, mix thoroughly, and gently clean your face. This is safe near the eyes.

2. Face Cleanser. Mix Macadamia oil and castor oil in equal proportions and use as a regular face cleanser in the evenings. This is a great natural remedy to cleanse the face and protect it from acne.

3. Macadamia Oil affects deeper layers of the skin, as well as strengthens, moisturizes, and renews them. Consider using it for baby massages, and to remove stretch marks from pregnancy.

4. Macadamia Oil for Nails. Macadamia oil is a great tool in the winter when the skin around the nail cuticles split. Treat the base of the nails with this oil to make it easier to remove the skin tags. Add a little oil in a bowl or cup, warm to your desired temperature, and soak your fingertips for 5 minutes. This procedure will make your nails healthy and beautiful. Repeat once a week.

Essential Oils and their Health Benefits

Accept the abundance of plants, aromatic herbs, and blossoms as a gift of nature and you will feel the aura of its special care.
— Belinda Grant Viagas. Holistic health care.

If you've enjoyed the scent of a rose, you have most probably experienced the aromatic qualities of essential oils. These naturally occurring, volatile, aromatic compounds are found in the seeds, bark, stems, roots, flowers, and other parts of plants. Essential oils give plants their distinctive smells, while they also help to protect them and play a role in plant pollination. Essential oils can be used for a wide range of emotional and physical applications either as single essential oils or in blends, depending on user experience and the desired benefit. Essential oils are used in aromatherapy which is considered an alternative medicine.

Essential oils are a hydrophobic fluid formed from aromatic plant compounds. They are used for perfumes, soaps, cosmetics, foods, beverages, incense, and home cleaning products. Essential oils are a natural, non-chemical alternative to traditional cosmetics. They evaporate to spread their aroma and to cleanse the air. Essential oils may be applied directly onto the skin, and are often used for massage, bathing, or skin care.

Lavender Essential Oil. Lavender's (Lavandula angustifolia) antibacterial properties help to combat infections from microbes, so lavender essential oil is often applied to natural cleansing and body washing products. Lavender oil has a mild aroma. Pouring lavender oil into a hot bath not only calms the nervous system but also improves the quality of sleep.

Rose Oil. Rose (Rosa damascena). It is best to collect rose oils made in Bulgaria or Turkey, as they will be of the highest quality. These softly distilled oils do not have a very strong smell and are used as oils for perfume production. Rose oil is also commonly used in aromatherapy.

Pine Essential Oil. Pine (Pinus sylvestris) has a bitter odor. This oil has antiseptic, antibacterial, and pain-reducing properties. It is also popular in holistic medicine.

Peppermint essential oil. Peppermint (Mentha piperita) is a hybrid species of spearmint and watermint (Mentha aquatica). Peppermint oil gives a cooling sensation and has a calming effect on the body. It can relieve sore muscles when used topically. It also has antimicrobial properties and can help freshen bad breath and soothe digestive issues. Peppermint oil can cause some side effects including heartburn and allergic reactions.

Bergamot essential oil. Bergamot (*Citrus aurantium var* or *Citrus bergamia*). Bergamot is a tropical citrus fruit whose seeds are used to extract the bergamot oil. The oil has a very sweet smell and several medicinal and industrial uses.

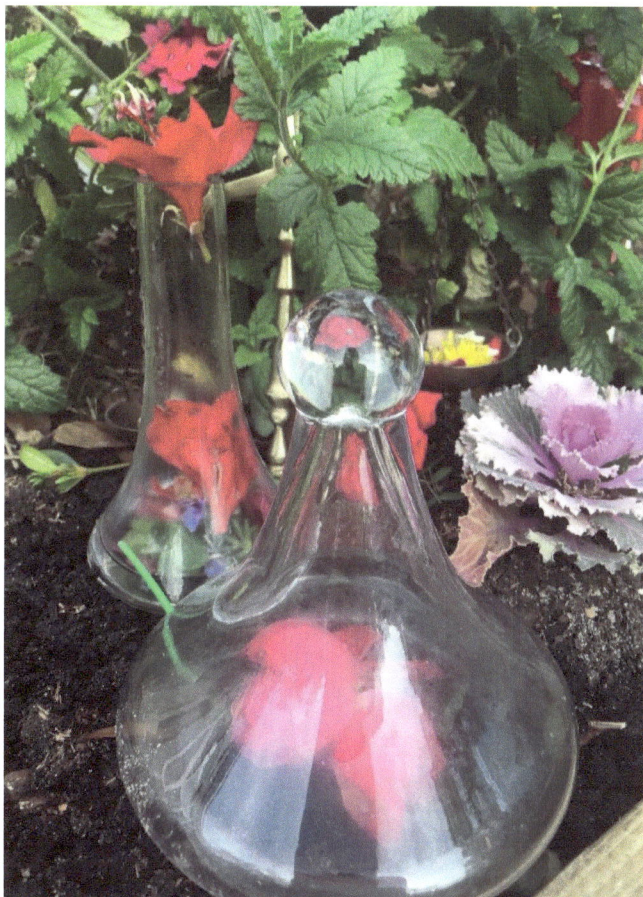

Chapter 14

FOLK MEDICINE ADVICE

The first duty of the physician is to educate the masses not to take medicine.
Sir William Osler, 1849-1919, Canadian physician.

If your eyes get tired due to spending too many hours at the computer, place a warm chamomile tea bags over the eyes, leave it there for 15-20 minutes. Visual disturbances can be helped with eating carrots or drinking carrot juice.

If your eyes are tired, or suppurate, wash them with a water and honey solution. To make this solution, add one teaspoon of raw honey in one glass of warm boiled water, stir well, and wash.

If you have a sore throat, use the following mixture: add one teaspoon of honey to a glass of hot milk in the evening before bedtime and again in the morning before eating. If you feel hoarse, your vocal cords will recover if you place a warm compress of steamed potatoes on the neck.

To cure bronchitis, try drinking a cup of tea in the evening: add to a cup of hot water 2-3 teaspoons of honey, a little lemon juice, and 2-3 teaspoons of rum.

If you catch a cold, or have bronchial asthma, rub your chest with garlic sauce mixed with butter.

For the cough of bronchitis, drink two tablespoons of a 1:1 mixture of black radish juice mixed with honey 15-20 minutes before meals.

Home remedy for bronchitis: mix five, small, finely chopped garlic cloves in 1 glass of raw milk and drink during the daytime.

When you feel that your nose is stuffed, you should first heat your feet in water mixed with salt or mustard powder. Also hot tea helps.

If you feel hoarse after a cold or cough, drink hot milk with honey. A hot bath will help to warm up your feet. Another aid is a warm compress to ease your neck tension.

If you have a persistent cough or suffer from bronchitis, drink 300g (7 oz.) of honey mixed with 0.5 glass of water and two large aloe vera leaves. To extract the aloe vera pulp, cut along the broad center of a leaf of aloe vera and scoop out the juice with a spoon and grind it. Mix the three ingredients and store the concoction in a cool place. It is recommended to drink one tablespoon three times a day.

If you catch a cold, eat more garlic and onion as they have strong bactericidal properties. Garlic reduces cholesterol in the blood and protects against infections.

Try hot milk with boiled garlic if you have a cough.

Garlic is **not recommended** for use in cases of gastritis or gastric ulcers.

Coughs can be reduced by using cherry, cranberry, or blackcurrant juice with honey. An apple decoction or tea also helps considerably.

If you have chronic bronchitis, take 500ml of wine, add the gel taken from four large, washed aloe vera leaves. Mix the gel with the wine and keep for 4 days. Dosage is one teaspoon 3 times a day.

To soothe a cough or ease a cold in spring, drink birch sap or maple juice with milk. You can also drink turnip juice with honey.

If you have a lack of appetite, exhaustion, coughing, abdominal pain, or skin infections, eat 2-3 slices of garlic per day, best with a few teaspoons of apple purée after meals.

Raw bee-pitch can be used to cure bed sores, ulcers, or burns.

Upper respiratory cataract: inhale the steam of just-cooked, mashed potatoes.

Fatigue will lessen and your well-being will improve if you take a bath in salted water or use Epsom salt. (A few handfuls of salt for one bath.)

You will avoid scurvy by eating pickled cabbages, green onions, and lemons.

Strengthening the Body and Preventing the Flu

1. Germinated wheat or barley grains strengthen the body. Soak the grains in water for 10 hours, cover with a damp gauze, and wait until the wheat germs are 1 mm high. Next, grind, mix with honey, raisins, and dried plums, and eat 1 spoon of this mixture 3 times a day.

2. Hawthorn tea with honey strengthens the body and protects against colds. This tea is prepared as follows: Soak hawthorn fruit in cold water for several hours, then grind it and add two tablespoons of dried hawthorn fruit to 200 ml of water. Heat until it boils. Once boiling, filter immediately and drink hot.

3. If you are feeling the first signs of influenza, peel a small onion, grate it, and spread the mass on a few layers of folded bandage. Put this compress on your nostrils and keep it there for about 10 minutes. Repeat this process 3 times a day. Before applying the compress, spread the nostrils with oil. It is also possible to pour the onion juice directly into the nose, but only after it is diluted with water or a solution of honey and water in a proportion of 1:5 or 1:10.

4. In order to feel better in the morning, take a nighttime drink of hot apple juice (like tea). Apple juice has a large concentration of pectin, which activates intestinal bacteria and eliminates viral toxins from the body faster. The recipe can be strengthened if you add thinly-cut orange peel, Ceylon cinnamon sticks, and 2-3 cloves (the spice) into 1 liter of warm juice. Cook on a low heat for about 20 minutes (Do not let it brew, as juice should only be hot).

5. Drink raspberry or blackberry juice if you have a cold, fever, or get hoarse. A wonderful tea made from dried raspberry berries and raspberry sticks helps to get rid of colds, fevers, or the flu (add two to three tablespoons of dried berries to one glass of boiling water). Drink 2-3 glasses of hot tea an hour before going to bed. In addition, cover yourself with something warm, and sweat freely.

6. If you have a blocked nose, take a hot, steamy bath and drink hot herbal tea with lemon and honey.

Use a mixture of garlic, honey, and lemon to strengthen the body. It is best to make a large batch that comprises 1 kg of honey, 10 lemons (rinsed well and grated), and 10 heads of garlic (cleaned and ground). Mix all the ingredients together and pour into a jar. Close the jar tightly and store it for a week in a cold place. Take 1-2 teaspoons each morning before meals.

Eating fish will help give you extra strength. Fish is especially rich in potassium salts, magnesium, phosphorus, and sodium. Try to eat fish soup twice a week.

If the body is weakened following illness, eat warm chicken broth cooked from organic chicken. When cooking the broth, eat a few leaves of parsley and pasta. This broth will help you regain strength.

Liver-friendly Nutrition

You must avoid eating foods that contain a lot of sugar, salt, or fat to prevent liver damage or disturb the functioning of the liver. In order to help clean the liver, which is a very important part of the body, it is necessary to eat only vegetarian food one day per month. Drinking the juice of one lemon greatly improves the functioning of the bile.

When feeling a heavy liver, it is recommended to drink infusions and cleavages of dill, sage, or dandelion grass, all of which improve the activity of this organ. Also, mineral water, fresh fruit, and vegetable juice all have major health benefits for the liver. Smoked or fatty meats, pastries, cakes, biscuits, chocolates, cocoa, canned meat, and pickled and salted products should also be avoided.

One of the best ways to treat the liver is by drinking fresh vegetable juice. Mix 210 ml of carrot juice, 150 ml of celery juice, and 60 ml of parsley. If inflammation develops in the liver, mix 40 g of dried marigold blossoms with 1 liter of boiling water. Drink the infusion 3 times a day.

Osteoporosis

If you have osteoporosis, drink kefir or buttermilk regularly. You can also eat curd, cheese, or yogurt. There is a great deal of calcium in fish, especially in salmon, while high concentrations are also present in vegetable food, soybeans, sunflower and sesame seeds, nuts, spinach, onions, and parsley.

To help keep strong bones, not only contain calcium but also magnesium and vitamin D are necessary. Plenty of magnesium is found in pineapples, bananas, parsley, dill, and potatoes (especially fried). Vitamin D is also produced by skin exposure to direct sunlight, and also found in wild fish.

Unstable Arterial Pressure

If you have hypertension, 140/90 or above, you should follow a specific diet that mainly comprises foods rich in potassium and calcium. You should also eat less salt and drink hawthorn decoctions and infusions.

In addition, you should stay physically active and do a daily meditation, such as imagining nice views, and control your emotions. Foods containing large amounts of salt increase the blood pressure, as do some cheeses and canned foods.

Recommendations for low arterial pressure

Drinking more liquids, coffee, and strong tea is essential. Wading in water or walking barefoot on the grass and snow is great for the whole body. Drying yourself with a damp towel is also a great way to train the blood vessels.
In the morning, eat 3 tablespoons of oat flakes soaked in a glass of cool milk mixed with 1 teaspoon of honey.

Atherosclerosis

Apple juice protects against atherosclerosis, strengthens the nervous system, and improves memory.

Recipe: Cranberries and garlic both protect against atherosclerosis.
Ingredients: 1/2 kg cranberries, 150g garlic, and 1kg of raw honey.
Preparation: Crush the cranberries and grind the garlic. Add them to 1kg of raw honey, mix, and store at room temperature. After two days, eat 1 teaspoon in the morning and 3 times a day 15-20 minutes before meals.

If you have hypertension and atherosclerosis, eat 2-3 small garlic cloves with an apple after meals.

Cabbages regulate metabolism and protect against atherosclerosis. They are suitable for gastritis with reduced acidity and intestinal inflammation.

Make dishes with eggplants if you have atherosclerosis. Eggplants also improve the functioning of the heart.

Preventing a Stroke

One of the most effective methods of stroke prevention is to follow a diet rich in antioxidants. Studies on over 37,000 women in Sweden over the course of eleven years have shown that participants with a high antioxidant diet were 17 percent less likely to suffer from strokes than those with a lack of antioxidants in their diet.
It has been found that stroke cases are significantly reduced when following a healthy diet containing plenty of fruits, vegetables, whole-grain foods, dark chocolate, and tea. This also helps to avoid being overweight. Being active and avoiding smoking are the most effective ways to avoid strokes.

The State Pathology Center of the University of Vilnius, Lithuania, advises a method to prevent a stroke using young pine cones. The pine cones improve the condition of the blood vessels of the head, increase their elasticity and tone, reduce blood pressure and stop brain tissue loss even after the stroke. Young, green pine cones need to be collected at the end of the summer. To a liter glass jar full of pine cones, fill with vodka up to the top and place it in a dark place for a couple of weeks, periodically shaking, until the liquid becomes a dark amber color. Then, add a tablespoon of apple cider vinegar. Mix it up, drain, and store in a dark place. Before bedtime, add 1 teaspoon of solution to a cup of hot tea and flavor with honey. When used at very high doses, pine preparations can cause stomach inflammation and headache.

From time to time, eat a mixture of healthy products. Such valuable health foods include 1 teaspoon of honey, 1 grated apple, and 1 small handful of peanuts or pumpkin seeds with lemon juice.

Folk medical advice to clean the blood vessels

1. Grate 1 lemon and add to ground garlic. Add this mix to 1.5 glasses of cool, boiled water. Keep at room temperature for 4 days and filter. Drink 1 teaspoon daily before meals, especially in autumn, winter, and spring.

2. Mix 1 cup of shelled walnuts with ½ cup of dried apricots, ½ cup of raisins and 2 unpeeled lemons. Pour all the ingredients into a meat grinder. Add 300 g (7 oz) of honey, grind until smooth, and store the mixture in a refrigerator. Take 1-2 teaspoons a day.

3. **Ingredients**: ½ liter (500ml) of vodka (as pure as possible), ½ liter (1 pound) of honey, ½ liter (1 pound) of crushed cranberries, and 2 lemons.
Preparation: Crush or grind the cranberries and add 2 finely chopped lemons with their peels. Mix all ingredients with honey and pour the vodka into a large jar. Close the jar and store it for 10 days in a dark place at room temperature. After 10 days, when the mixture has had enough time to ferment, consume 3 teaspoons on wakening. Remember to wait about 20 minutes before starting to eat breakfast. Duration: 3 months.

Hawthorn decoctions with honey help to ease heart pain.
Pour 500 ml boiling water over 1 tablespoon of dried fruit. Cover for 15-20 minutes, add 2 teaspoons of honey, and drink the decoction. Hawthorn decoctions are especially effective during the coldest months of the year.

With ischemic heart disease, it is recommended to regularly consume a mixture of honey and garlic. To do this, clean 4 cloves of garlic, grind them, mix with 350 g (8 ounces) of fresh honey and leave for 10 days in a dark place. Take 1 teaspoon 3 times a day before meals.

Eating sunflower seeds supports the normal functioning of the cardiovascular system. 50 g of sunflower seeds satisfies the body's recommended daily intake of vitamin E

Insomnia

If you suffer from insomnia, muscle cramps (especially at night), weak memory, or reduced work capacity, you should eat 1 tablespoon of honey per day, in addition to lots of vegetables and fruits, especially apples and grapes or their juice.

If you suffer from insomnia, place some sliced onion on your neck. The Swiss often say that eating green onion before bedtime helps one to fall asleep early.

If you suffer from insomnia, a linen pillow filled with fresh hops will help you sleep better.

Valerian tablets or their drops will help to overcome insomnia and stress. Try taking one or two tablets before going to bed, or add a few drops to a teaspoon of sugar.

If it is hard to fall asleep and if your legs feel very cold, take a warm shower before going to bed, or make a warm bath for your legs and drink a glass of warm milk before bedtime.

Metabolism

To increase tone, improve metabolism, and heal respiratory diseases and lung diseases, open the windows to ventilate your room every morning. When doing this, try to breathe for 5 minutes by taking 4-5 deep breaths, followed by 5 smooth exhalations. Of course, it also greatly helps if you live in a village or in a seaside resort.

To alleviate symptoms of anemia and rheumatism, hazelnuts and honey are good remedial ingredients.

If you have anemia, drink fresh pomegranate, lemon, carrot, apple, juices and eat honey.

The Following Compresses Are Good for Swollen Eyelids

1. Put grated potatoes or chopped cucumber between two layers of gauze and place them on closed eyelids for half an hour. The swelling should disappear if you continue this procedure for two weeks.

2. Fill two small bags with dried chamomile blossoms or dried rose leaves. Before using, immerse the bag in hot water. After cooling, lay gently on your closed eyes. You can also make such compresses by boiling chamomile tea. After drinking tea, place cooled chamomile tea bags over your eyelids for half an hour.

3. Black tea reduces the swelling of the eyelids. Hold the wet tea bags on the eyelids for 15 minutes.

4. For dark circles, tired, and puffy eyes, grate 1 cucumber, smash ½ banana, mix all together, pour into an ice cube tray and freeze it. Take one ice cube each morning and move around eyes.

How to Avoid Gastrointestinal Diseases in Summer

Gastrointestinal malfunctions increase in summer. When this happens, the abdomen can suddenly start to hurt without reason, together with the onset of nausea and diarrhea. Although the symptoms of various diseases are similar, their causes may be different. "Dirty Hand" diseases are acute intestinal infections, manifested by nausea, vomiting, diarrhea, and often severe hemorrhage. We call these "dirty hand" diseases because they can become infected due to not washing the hands before eating and not following other hygiene rules. However, in general, their agents can spread through contaminated food and water, among other causes, such as the presence of flies on food. In order to avoid poisoning, a number of personal hygiene rules should be followed; namely, hand washing, precise washing of fresh fruits and vegetables, and eating only fresh high-quality food. If you experience symptoms of poisoning and start to feel nauseous but you cannot vomit, drink one teaspoon of baking soda in a glass of warm water, stir, and drink one sip at a time. After getting rid of the uncooked food you will feel much better. Following this, drink plenty of warm liquids and warm chamomile tea without sugar and refrain from eating until the next morning. In the morning, prepare a chicken broth and do not eat hard food until you get better.

Chamomile blossoms. The active substances contained in blossoms reduce inflammation. Therefore, they are particularly suitable for acute or chronic inflammation of the gastrointestinal mucosa. In addition, the preparations of chamomile blossoms effectively reduce bloating and spasms. It is recommended to drink chamomile tea if you are suffering from acute gastritis or when the stomach feels burned. Mix 2 teaspoons of chamomile blossoms poured with hot (not boiling) water and leave for 5-10 minutes. This tea is drunk warm and always before eating; moreover, it cannot be sweetened. If you suffer from inflammation of the large intestine, it is advisable to make an enema of chamomile blossom decoction on a daily basis. The repeated use of chamomile blossoms will eventually diminish its effectiveness.

For gastric or duodenal ulcers, you should eat small portions of liquid or pure food that is either stewed or cooked at room temperature 5-6 times a day. Use vegetable oils, which contain linoleic acid and can help to prevent ulcer exacerbation. Eat less rich food with fiber as this can irritate the damaged mucous membranes. Eat bananas, red beets, and parsley leaves, and drink juices made from white cabbage, carrots, and cucumber. Drink at least 1 glass of warm herbal tea infusion daily. One should also stop drinking alcohol and coffee because these drinks stimulate the production of hydrochloric acid in the stomach. Cranberries treat gastritis and reduce the acidity. Such acidity will also decrease if you drink ½ a glass of fresh carrot juice in the morning before breakfast.

During ulcer flare ups, do not eat acid fruits and berries.

Reflux treatment by natural means.
It is advisable to drink a glass of warm water in the morning on an empty stomach. After this, wait for 10-15 minutes and eat breakfast. During the day, drink lots of water. Water raises the pH of the stomach and reduces the acidity.
In order to prevent reflux, here are some essential dietary rules:
1. In one serving, eat up to 300g of warm food.
2. Consume less food than you would typically eat, and refrain from eating fried, smoked, spicy, and salty foods.
3. Eat warm soup, fruits, and meat. In particular, try to eat foods that digest quickly.
4. Try to avoid taking on too much fluid during meals and immediately after eating.
5. After eating, try not to bend the body excessively. It is also important to not lift heavy items or lie horizontally.
6. Reduce or eliminate all flour and sugar products from your diet.
7. Stop smoking and drinking alcohol and coffee.

If you have a gnawing stomach pain, it is recommended to drink milk, mucous decoctions, and jelly pastes. Avoid eating fatty fish and meat, soft-boiled eggs, wheat semolina, rice porridges, and white bread. Refrain from eating sour food or dark bread. It is important not to overeat. Eat until you are almost full.

Eat raspberries to improve digestion or if you suffer from anemia or stomach pain. Eat blackcurrant berries and drink their juice if you have breakdowns in the stomach or the intestines. If you have digestion problems, drink apples or carrot juice. Fruit juices clear the digestive system and contain a lot of vitamins. A small glass of whey or sauerkraut juice before a meal is good for the digestive system.

An oatmeal decoction with honey boosts energy levels following a period of illness. Oat drinks with a jelly paste are suitable for people with stomach and intestinal diseases.

The Tibetans say that everyone who is over 40 years old should eat a few teaspoons of semolina wheat porridge every day. Semolina wheat porridge benefits the bones, muscles, stomach, and intestines.

Preventing Constipation

1. Linseed. The laxative sensation of the linseeds begins 2-3 days following consumption. It is recommended to eat 2 tablespoons of minced linseeds with 2 glasses of water in the morning and in the evening. To be more effective, mix the linseeds with fruit or honey.
2. Black plums and figs. Soak 3-5 black plums or figs in water. In the morning (before eating breakfast), consume the liquid and eat the fruits. The laxative effect will occur after 2-3 hours.
3. Potato juice is used for the treatment of constipation and ulcers of the digestive tract. This juice also softens stomach disorders and decreases gastric acid secretion. Drink 2-3 times a day with ½ a cup of fresh, green potato juice half an hour before a meal.
4. Kefir or buttermilk strengthens intestinal peristalsis. It is recommended to drink 2-3 glasses during the day.
5. For chronic bowel congestion prevention, eat 100-150 g of cooked beet or half a pumpkin on an empty stomach every day.

Diarrhea Prevention

If you have diarrhea, rice, rice porridge, or an oat flake decoction will ease your troubles. You can also drink chamomile or cumin tea, or eat dried blueberry berries. Apple puree helps constipation as well as acute and chronic inflammation of the large intestine, and other impaired bowel activity.

Flatulence can be reduced by biting cinnamon peel and parsley or by eating mints. Peppermint tea and dill help to relieve intestinal spasms and suppress bloating.

Urinary issues:

Eat watermelons in order to avoid biliary and ureteric stones and anemia.

Bladder irritation is effectively treated with the following tea: take 1 tablespoon of bearberry leaves (Uva Ursi), add 2 glasses of water and boil until one glass of decoction remains. Drink one glass 3 times a day.

Drink cranberry juice in order to avoid kidney stones. For treatment of sands and stones in the kidneys, it is necessary to drink at least 1.5-2 liters of liquids per day, such as boiled water, herbal tea, milk, cranberry juice, and fresh lemon juice. Before breakfast every morning, drink 1 glass of birch sap. Other stone treatment suggestions include consuming half a glass of red currant juice three times a day, eat pumpkins and melons, plums, apples, onions, dill, carrots, and sweet potatoes. Avoid salt and meat. Do not drink alcohol, avoid constipation and being overweight.

For urinary incontinence, pour a glass of boiling water over 1 tablespoon of dill seeds and store in a warm place (preferably put in a thermos). Consume the entire mixture over the course of 1 day.

If you have urinary incontinence at night, drink St. John's wort. Take one tablespoon 3 times a day.

Other miscellaneous suggestions

If you have anemia or low blood pressure, eat the liver of a large horned animal. Chop the liver meat finely and fry, but not completely. Alternatively, grind the liver in a meat grinder, make a meat pie, and eat 100 g every day.

To relieve arthritis, drink a glass of warm boiled water, 1 teaspoon of honey, and 2 teaspoons of organic apple cider vinegar. Drink once a day.

If you have a toothache, place a piece of onion on the affected tooth until you can see the dentist. Most people find that the pain usually goes away.

People who have a gland affliction, suck the crumbs of bees' pitch (several times a day) until the swelling reduces. You can also wear amber necklaces or eat cedar nuts.

If you want to eliminate pigmentary stains on your face, it is recommended to rub the stain with the following liquid at night: 3 parts of fresh unpasteurized milk and 1 part of pure alcohol.

If you have stretch marks on your belly, it might help to rub with 1 leave aloe vera gel, mixed with 1 tablespoon coconut oil. The stretch marks should disappear after 3 months.

Onion juice covered with a gauze cleanses and heals suppurating wounds and ulcers.

Raw bee pitch is used for the treatment of warts, corns, and long-lasting wounds and burns.

If you have abscesses or infected wounds, cover these areas with a bandage greased with honey.

If you have stomach, intestinal, or cardiovascular diseases or metabolism disorders, eat tomatoes.

If you have liver, kidney diseases, gastritis, or intestinal inflammation, do not use radishes.

The Humble Potato

Raw potatoes have a high level of potassium, niacin, and vitamin C. It's a great food to help the following eight ailments.
1. Stomach disorders, ulcers, and gastritis can be mitigated by drinking potato juice.
2. When drinking potato juice, the antioxidants present in the juice can help to reduce cholesterol.
3. Drinking 1-2 teaspoons of potato juice before each meal can help to relieve symptoms of arthritis. As an alternative, boil the potato peelings for 3-5 minutes, strain off the starch, and drink this liquid when it cools down. Repeat four times a day to reduce pain and inflammation.
4. Rub grated potatoes into the skin. The skin will be hydrated and will absorb a lot of nutrients.
5. If you have a headache, rounded, chopped potatoes can help. If you have a chronic headache, try drinking ¼ cup of potato juice before eating.
6. You will improve the liver and gallbladder if you boil potato peels with a cup of water. Drain off the starch and drink this liquid when it cools down.
7. To prevent irritation and itchiness from insect bites, put slices of raw potato on your irritated skin.
8. Potatoes can also help to fight against certain types of cancers.

Making potato juice is very simple. Cut the potatoes into small cubes and juice them in a blender. Once the desired consistency has been obtained, drink the juice.

Tissue Restoration

Certain fruits contain ingredients that help maintain resistant and durable tissues. Once a year for a month and a half have a nightly bedtime snack of 1 dried fig, 5 dried apricots, and 1 dried black plum. These fruits contain substances that restore the tissues that comprise the intervertebral discs. By reinforcing these tissues, the vertebrae can return to their original position without correction. The substances required are not available in separate fruits; thus, they can only be obtained by mixing them.

Curd and Oil

Dr. Johanna Budwig was one of the leading European researchers of cancer biochemistry. She was born in 1908 and died at the age of 95 years. During her lifetime, she was nominated seven times for the Nobel Prize for special merits in the treatment of cancer. One of her major discoveries was the "Budwig protocol."

Linseed oil has a high content of OMEGA-3 fatty acids. It is easily digestible and does not cause allergies. Curd contains high levels of glycoproteins. The combination of curd and linseed oil makes the fatty acids water-soluble and easily absorbed by the body. The use of this combination, later called the "Budwig Protocol", has proven its therapeutic value in the treatment of cancer, and also been found useful for treating other conditions, such as heart attacks, atherosclerosis, liver function disorders, arthritis, and skin eczema. A curd and linseed diet is beneficial for everyone.

To prepare this food, combine one part organic, cold pressed flaxseed oil with two parts of curd on a daily basis. Blend it then grind your preferred amount of flaxseeds to add to the mix for texture and fiber. Mix the ground flaxseeds into puree and you are ready to eat. Dr. Budwig recommended eating a mixture with fresh fruit to make it even healthier. It should be noted that linseed oil is perishable. When you buy it at a store, look at the bottling date. If the linseed oil was bottled more than a month previously, it will be 100% corrupted, even if the expiration date is six months. Store-bought oil should be kept in the refrigerator. Oil cannot be stored in light or heat because it gets bitter and unusable.

How to Defeat Sinusitis

1. Peel and wash a slice of garlic, chop it with a thin grater, and mix it with a piece of butter that is the same size or a little bigger than the garlic slice. (Be careful not to add too much garlic, otherwise the grease can be too strong and burn the skin). In the evening, massage the neck and nose with this grease, as well as any other areas where purulent excreta are accumulated when you have sinusitis. Smooth your feet with this grease, wait until they dry, and sleep in a bed with warm socks. In the morning, cook some potatoes, cover your head with a thick towel, and breathe in their steam for about 10-15 minutes. After the first procedure, you will find that a large amount of mucus will be released from

the sinuses. You will also find that pain will decrease and your body temperature will begin to stabilize. This procedure can be repeated several times.

2. Add 3-5 chopped garlic cloves to boiled water. Lean over the steaming pot, cover your head with a towel and breathe deeply.

3. Grind in a meat, or hand grinder strong smelling peppers, (red-chili pepper, cayenne, jalapeno) and inhale. (Keep away from eyes).

3. Rub a trimmed onion into a few pieces of gauze. Place the gauze into each nostril and breathe in the scent.

Clearing Body Toxins

If you want to be healthy, every morning consume a cup of warm boiled water mixed with one teaspoon of honey pressed together with the same amount of lemon juice half an hour before breakfast. This will clear the body from toxins.

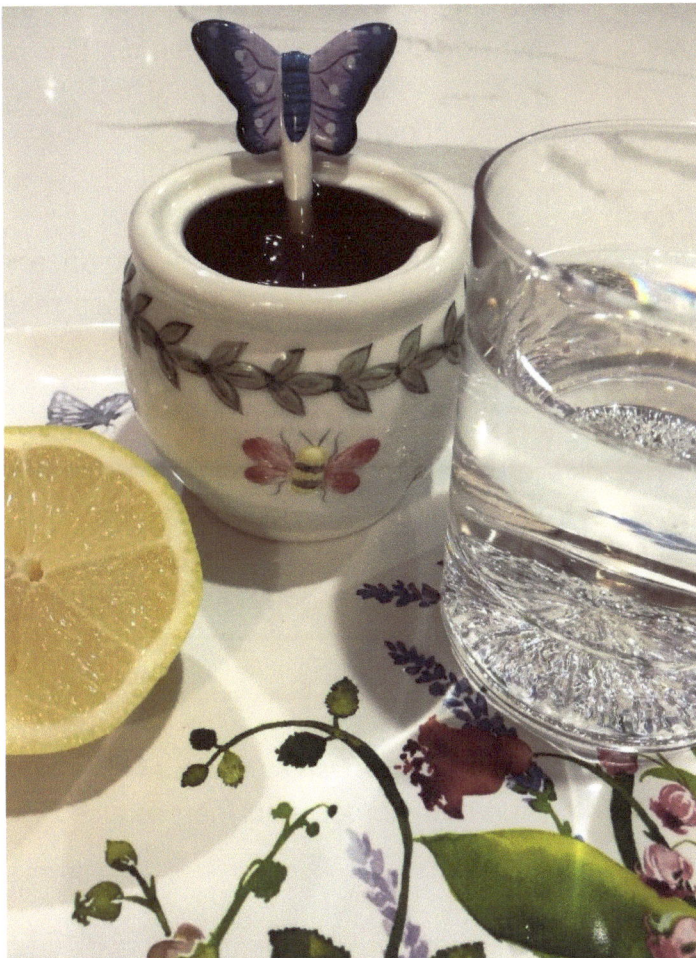

When it comes to diseases, most of them are easier to prevent than cure. One of the most important factors is a healthy diet. Overheated fats found in fried meat, fish, cakes, etc. are extremely dangerous for the blood vessels. These fats accumulate on the walls of the blood vessels and become cholesterol plaques, which eventually narrow the opening of blood vessels and form blood clots.

Chapter 15

THE SECRETS OF LONGEVITY

Keep close to Nature's heart...and break clear away once in a while, and climb a mountain, or spend a week in the woods. Wash your spirit clean.
— John Muir, 1838-1914.

How to live a longer life

These techniques prove that Americans can live up to 80, 90, and even 100 years-old and beyond.

1. Obtain the right amount of vitamin D.
Vitamin D is necessary for bone health, but too much can cause various problems, such as kidney stones. Vitamin D is produced by exposure to the sun, depending on your skin coloration, about 15 minutes a day on bare arms is sufficient. Too much exposure to the sun creates a risk of developing skin cancer. Your doctor can test your vitamin D level and tell you if you need supplements. Research from Copenhagen University has shown the ideal vitamin content to be between 50 and 100 nmol per liter of blood.

2. Limit the use of NSAID pain relief drugs.
Regular use of these drugs, such as Ibuprofen and naproxen, including Advil, Motrin, and Aleve, increase the risk of having a heart attack or stroke. Limit your use of pain relief medicine to short periods.

3. Sleep at least eight hours.
Constant sleep for six hours or less increases the possibility of getting a heart attack or stroke. It is important to close the curtains before sleeping in order to maintain darkness. Keeping the room temperature between 60-67F degrees helps sleep. It is also important to work out every day and to avoid looking at electronic screens one hour before you go to sleep. If your mattress is more than ten years old, replace it.

4. To marry or not to marry?
A happy marriage helps you to live a longer life. A 2014 study from students at New York University's Langone Medical Center found that married women and men reduced the likelihood of contracting a cardiovascular disease by 5%.

5. Eat fully ripened fruit.
Green bananas have less fiber and are rich in tannins, which can harden laxatives. Completely ripe blueberries and fully mature pears have more antioxidants which fight against the diseases. Watermelons of a deep red color have more lycopene and antioxidants which can reduce the likelihood of cancer and heart disease.

6. Frozen fruits or vegetables are good for you.
Frozen fruits and vegetables perfectly preserve nutrients. British scientists have found that fruit you consume after three days may lose many nutrients. Frozen blueberries retain more vitamin C than freshly picked ones.

7. Minimize the use of sugar.
Excessive use of sugar increases blood sugar levels, leading to a threefold increased risk of heart and cardiovascular diseases. The American Heart Association recommends that women should limit their daily sugar dose to no more than 6 teaspoons (25g), and men no more than 9 teaspoons (36g).

8. Eat whole grain foods.
Eating three or more full grains every day can help prevent many diseases, according to a 2016 Harvard University TH Chan School of Public Health study. It is recommended to eat oatmeal, brown rice, barley and other cereals in the morning.

9. Insert spices into the food.
Eating chili pepper can prolong your life. By eating chili peppers, the body can produce more endorphins that reduce pain and inflammation.

10. Drink water.
Studies from researchers at the University of Illinois have found that people who drink more water eat less, which allows them to reduce weight. Drinking plenty of water reduces the risk of developing bladder and colon disease, and also allows for optimal renal functioning.

11. Eat less.
The average Japanese person stops eating when they feel 80% full. A National Institutes of Health study found that cutting calories leads to reduced blood pressure and cholesterol. .When cooking or ordering food out, purposely choose small portions.

12. Stop eating earlier in the evening.
Late night eating soon before going to bed increases your risk of developing heart disease and accumulating body fat.

13. Eat more vegetables.
A study on 73,000 adults who ate vegetables, fish, eggs, and dairy products had a longer life expectancy than those who ate lots of meat and little vegetables.

14. Eat to the Greeks.
The Mediterranean diet is filled with fruits, vegetables, nuts, and fish. Harvard researchers in 2014 found that this diet helped people live a longer and healthier life.

15. Live as an Amish.
Research from the University of Maryland has shown that the Amish visited hospitals at a lower rate than other populations. This is attributed to factors such as not smoking or drinking alcohol, keeping physically active, respecting their social structure, and staying involved in their families and in the community affairs.

16. Drink less alcohol.
More than one drink in the day for women and two drinks for men leads to a shorter lifespan. Even for red wine, one can reduce the amount of alcohol by using a white wine glass, which is narrower.

17. Visit mountains.
If there is a possibility to live in the mountains, do it! According to the University of Colorado and the Harvard School of Global Health, humans live longer by living in the mountains. It is believed that the body adapts to the lower oxygen content found at higher altitudes. In this way, being in the mountains can help strengthen both heart and blood circulation, while it also eases stress.

18. Eat nuts.
European studies have shown that eating nuts daily can reduce the risk of health problems by up to 23%, as well as the avoidance of heart disease, cancer, and respiratory diseases. This excludes peanuts, which are legumes and not nuts.

19. Find yourself an intriguing hobby.
Any activity that stimulates your mind will increase your lifespan. Examples include sports, pet care, dancing, games, astronomy, and photography.

20. Plan out your day.
Get up early in the morning and think of your activities for the day. It is important to have goals in your day.

21. Have your faith.
Go at least once a week to church and take part in church activities such as choir.

22. Go on vacation.
Those who don't vacation have a higher probability of developing coronary artery disease and heart attacks. You should take leave at least twice a year.

23. Make friends with four-legged creatures.
Four-legged friends help reduce anxiety, lower blood pressure, and reduce the chance of having a heart attack. According to the American Heart Association, dog owners are more active people and have less stress.

24. Watch comedy shows and movies.
Laughter is a good medicine to help cope with stress, enhance the immune system to relieve pain, and adjust the blood flow to the brain. Laughter also boosts the blood vessels when exercising, according to the University of Maryland School of Medicine in Baltimore.

25. Communicate.
Studies have shown that loneliness increases the risk of death by 45%, by reducing the immune system, increasing the blood pressure, and increasing risk of heart attacks and strokes. Keep in touch with friends, family, and people. A 2016 study from the University of California, San Diego, found that people who interact through Facebook live longer.

26. Read.
Read newspapers, magazines, and books. Try to spend at least half an hour reading each day.

27. Choose to walk up and down the stairs when possible.
Spending half an hour a day burning calories by walking benefits the brain, heart, skin, and mood, and improves metabolism.

28.Maintain contact with grandchildren.
Maintaining regular contact with one's grandchildren will help you to remain mentally and physically active.

The Japanese recommend the following:

1. Drink purified water and you will stay healthy and active.
2. Do not drink coffee more than once a day.
3. Take tablets with room temperature water, rather than cold.
4. Do not eat after 5 pm.
5. Eat a minimum amount of fatty foods.
6. Drink plenty of water in the morning and less in the evening.
7. Avoid fried foods. They have cholesterol and cancerogenic substances.
8. Give your brain work to do.
9. The best time to sleep is 10 pm - 6 am.
10. Send a message to those who care about you.
11. Do not hurry.
12. Restrict sugar use to one teaspoon a day.
13. Eat 500 grams of fresh vegetables daily. Consider a salad with fresh cabbage, beetroot, carrot, and turnip. Use oil rather than mayonnaise as dressing.
14. Pamper your body in a spa two or three times a month.
15. Take stewed foods three to four times a week. This juvenile-style broth retains more of the vitamins and minerals needed for your body.
16. Add sea cabbage to the menu. 500 grams a day will remove harmful substances from the body.
17. Carefully chew food to facilitate the work of your digestive organs.
18. Cook a fish soup twice or three times a week. Fish broth is rich in substances that prolong youth.
19. Find a hobby. Do not sit in front of the TV for more than an hour a day.
20. Say "No" to white bread. The Japanese do not eat white bread.
21. Spend more time outside. Have weekly outdoor picnics.
22. Accustom your body to the cold.
23. Drink 3-4 cups of green tea a day.
24. Move more.
25. Cure yourself of minor illnesses and seek professional medical help when needed.
26. Do not calumniate others. Say good or say nothing, often it is best to keep quiet.
27. Have water and cooked porridge on your breakfast table. They have minerals and keep you younger for longer.
28. Communicate.
29. Traditional Japanese home cooked meals tend to center around a main protein dish with several additional vegetables dishes to accompany it and is usually eaten with steamed rice, miso soup and pickles. They eat raw fish in sushi and sashimi, plus a lot of pickled, fermented and smoked foods. The main course can be fish, chicken, beef and pork. Switch beef and pork for fish and chicken breasts.

Important detail: The Chinese and Japanese drink hot tea while eating (not cold water or sodas).

An explanation for those who like to drink cold drinks during a meal.

Cold water reduces digestion of fatty foods because the fats in food thicken with cold drinks. When drinking hot drinks, oxygen is more slowly released into the fat and food is better digested in the intestines than drinking cold drinks. As a result, less fat accumulates under the skin and the likelihood of cancer is reduced by ten times.

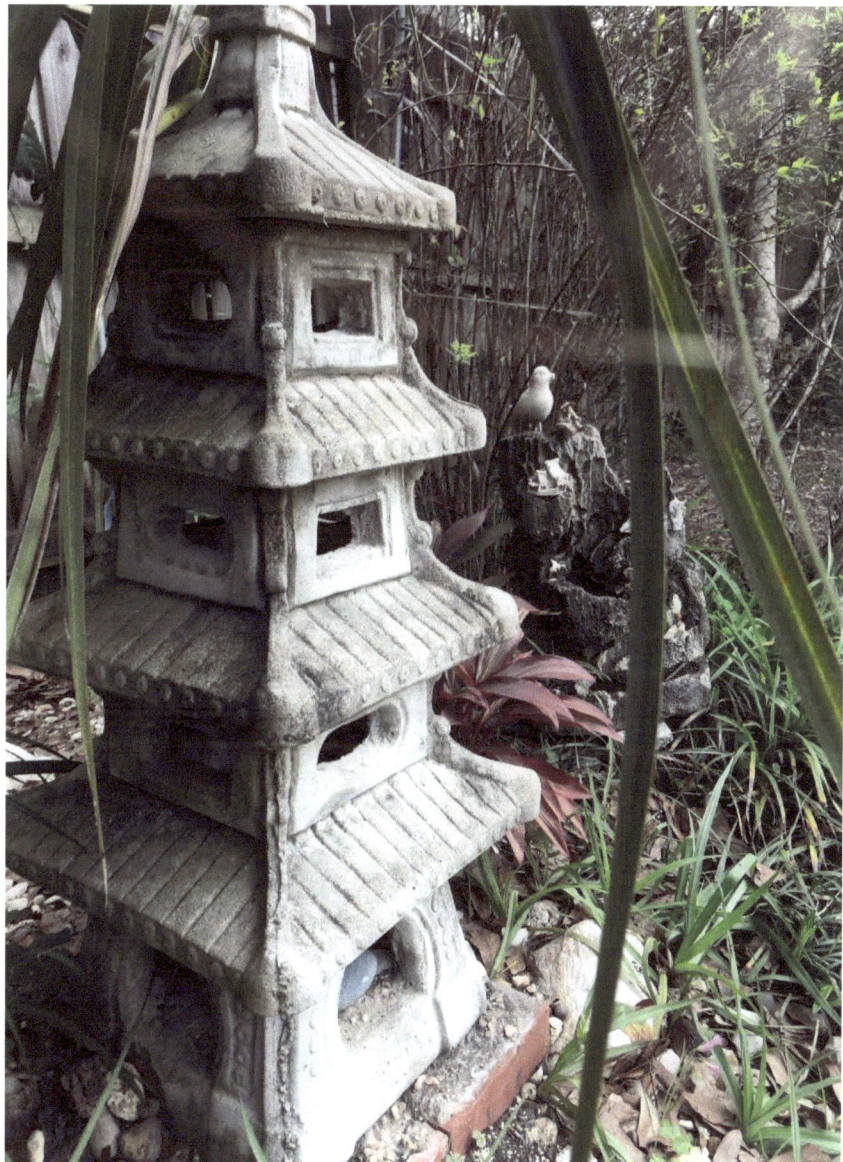

MOUNTAIN PEOPLE from the Caucasian Mountains recommend the following.

There are locations that are famous for the strength of the body and spirit. Why are they healthy and enchanting even when they are at an honorable age? Perhaps we can learn something from their longevity, especially since their advice is simple: they do not require much time or cost, and the effect is astounding.

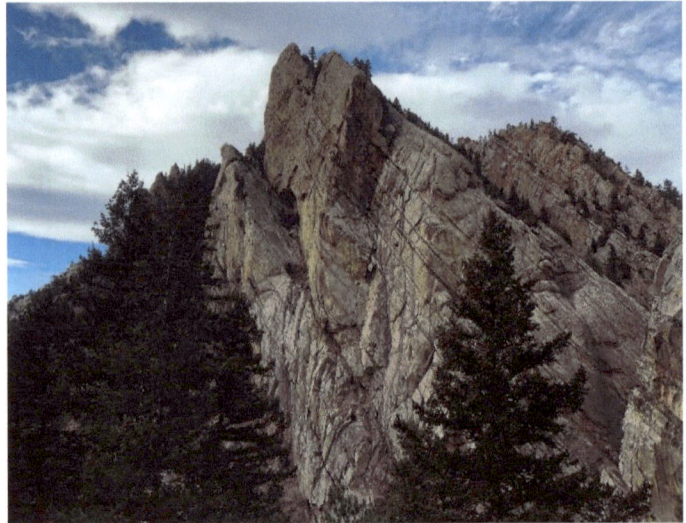

1. Animal Influences. Mountain people are always surrounded by dogs, horses, sheep, and other animals. The energy of animals is extremely useful to the human being. Caring for animals allows you to forget your loneliness and helps overcome depression.

2. Clothing: From ancient times, the Caucasian people have made their clothes from natural materials that support heat in the winter, absorb moisture in the summer, and cool the body. Like them, it is advisable to wear wool clothes in winter and cotton and linen clothes in summer. Scientists have established that clothing from these materials allows the body to maintain its normal energy and heat metabolism, thus preventing aging. Highly valuable clothing is knitted of wool and should be worn when you have bronchitis or inflammation of the lungs. If you suffer from radiculitis or kidney disease, gird yourself with a wide belt.

3. God's Food. Mountain people mostly eat fresh fruits, vegetables, greens, nuts, and low-fat dairy products. Western people often eat meat, but meat dishes should be limited. Caucasian people eat their traditional shashlik (shish-kabob) only during celebrations or festivities. When you do eat meat, choose oven-cooked or grilled for the fat to flow out. God's food for the mountain people are their drinks, kefir (sour milk-type drink) and ayran (a yogurt based drink). Not surprisingly, many doctors recommend kefir because it is absorbed and digested much better than milk. Kefir evokes the appetite, tones the nervous and cardiovascular systems, and suppresses rotting processes in the stomach and intestines. Ayran is just as powerful a drink. This product restores the microflora in the intestine, improves intestinal peristalsis, and helps in the treatment of dysbacteriosis.

Kefir Recipe: Add 3 tablespoons of water to a glass of sour milk, add salt (on the tip of the knife) and a few pieces of ice, and the life elixir is ready. Drink 2 glasses of kefir or ayran daily. Scientists have determined that life lengthens for 10 years if you use these products every day.

4. Wine. You can drink 50-100 ml of dry red wine to make your food more digestible. This protects against infections and strokes, oncological diseases, and it also helps in regulating the blood pressure.

5. Body Massage. Another secret to the health of the Caucasian people is that the active points of feet and palms and nerve endings are constantly stimulated. They wear soft shoes; thus, stones massage their feet. The grapes are picked by hand, pots of clay are often used to serve food, and the clay is very carefully soiled. Winemakers knead the berries with their legs—a specific massage that has a positive effect on the whole body.

6. Exercise. Take regular exercise every day and you will feel your body become more flexible. You will feel you are younger and have more energy.
a)   A good exercise is a balance practice: Lay a six-foot strap on the floor and try walking its length without stepping off.
b)   Take a large flat-bottom bowl or plastic storage box and add a one-inch layer of smooth stones or river gravel. Step in and out of it barefoot two or three times a day for at least 10 minutes. For an added treat, add water to give the impression of being in a water stream. When drying your feet, give them a massage and perhaps some healing lotion. You may want to advance to larger stones over time. As an alternative, wade in the fresh dew after getting up in the morning, if you have the opportunity. Your feet will be well-massaged and your body will be hardened.
c)   Everybody admires the gait of the Caucasian women. Since childhood, Caucasian women are accustomed to carrying jugs of wine or water on their heads, and they walk straight all the time with proudly raised heads. Such a walk is both beautiful and healthy for the backbone and thus for the whole body. To practice such posture, balance a book on your head and walk around your room. Initially, do the exercise for 3 minutes and try to work your way up to 10 minutes or more.

7. Who gets up early, never regrets.
The Caucasians get up early in order to have time to finish their work. It is said that the one who does not see the rising sun, does not see a new day. Because death often occurs just before sunrise, those who rise early may delay their own deaths. Getting up early is healthy. In order to maintain high spirits, you must go to bed by 10 p.m. and get up at 6 a.m.

8. Bee's pitch. The main medicine for the Caucasian mountain people is not pills or drops but a pitch. They claim that this bee product can cure any disease. In cases of influenza, angina, stomach aches, pain in the teeth or gums, or if you have a gastric ulcer, they recommend holding a pea-sized pitch piece under the tongue for 4-6 hours (if possible longer) per day. Even if you swallow, it's not harmful and the body will take what it needs. If you suffer from rheumatism, arthritis, or osteochondrosis, the pitch can be warmed up and placed on the painful area. Pitch ointment is applied to treat skin eczema.

Bee Pitch Recipe: Warm 100 g of Vaseline until boiling, cool until 50-60°C, add a teaspoon of pitch mixture, and warm up to 70-80°C. Mix it with a wooden rod until the pitch is dissolved. Filter through 4 layers of gauze and close the bowl with the mixture. Once cooled, apply the mixture on painful spots.

Aqueous Pitch Recipe: This pitch is useful to drink when you have stomach and gastrointestinal tract diseases. Dissolve 20 g of pitch in 200 ml of water and steam for 10-15 minutes. Cool for 1 hour and mix with a glass rod from time to time. Filter, store in a cool place, and take a spoonful 3 times a day before eating. If you suffer from angina, laryngitis, pharyngitis, stomatitis, or periodontitis. you can rinse your mouth in this solution diluted with water 1:1.

Spiritual Pitch Recipe. This solution is the elixir of youth. It cleanses the body perfectly, eliminates waste and toxins, strengthens immunity, and delays senility. Mix 1 part of the pitch with 10 parts of 70% spirits, close tightly, and store for 3 days, occasionally stirring. Then, filter through one layer of gauze. Add 20-30 drops to ½ glass of milk or water and drink three times a day 1-1.5 hours before a meal.

9. A glimpse of enlightenment.
As one long-lived Abkhaz person once said, "*We are healthy because there is peace in our soul. Anger and jealousy impede life. You do not need to envy anyone, and keep away from those who are jealous of you.*"
Mountain inhabitants avoid noise. The most important thing is to learn how to rest. No matter how busy you are, take an hour or a half hour to yourself. During this time, do what you like most, i.e., read a book, watch a movie, or go for a walk. If possible, walk to work. And if you are working far away, take two or three stops and go on foot. Try to walk when you return from work. At least a half-hour spent walking is very helpful. In addition, take exercise a few times a day. "Looking to eternity" is what the Caucasian people say when looking at the world from their high mountains. So, sit straight, relax, and look at infinity. It does not matter what you see before yourself—whether a wall, a burning fire, or a peaceful tree, just look as if you look at the infinite distance.

According to a Caucasian proverb, "*If your character does not rest, you will not live for a long time.*" Caucasian people think that no matter how hard life is, it is worthy of love; thus, you only need to be curious, calm, and good.

10. Help others feel better. A modern person is unlikely to be able to learn from the long-lived to be calm and untangled. However, nowadays, when there are so many stressful situations, and when you are psychologically tired, it is very important for the nervous system to be healthy. Try not to keep anger in yourself; instead, learn to forgive your offenders and yourself. Try to treat people as you would expect them to do with you so that there is no reason to hurt them. Good people live longer. Recent scientific research has found that people who help others feel better than those who are locked up in their labyrinth of worries. The inhabitants of the Caucasus are known for being very hospitable and generous people.

Thus, one of the secrets of longevity is to give more, not take. It is a proven fact that knowing that you are in need prolongs life. If you don't have money to buy an expensive gift for your friends, no problem. If you are away, bring your friends an interesting, even a cheap souvenir, and send a postcard. It will bring joy. Always feel grateful for a good word, encouragement, or good work done for you.

Moreover, do not bolt yourself in your world, help people as much as you can. If at least one person seems grateful, you will be happy. Never give up because of others' pessimism. Strive for high goals, expand your thinking, and do not give in to the absurd idea that high expectations are dangerous. Great hopes will revitalize your life. Fulfill your high goals and think broadly.

If you want to achieve something and feel that you will not succeed, just imagine Michelangelo, who lived five hundred years ago, who was still painting, gouging, and writing at the age of eighty-nine.

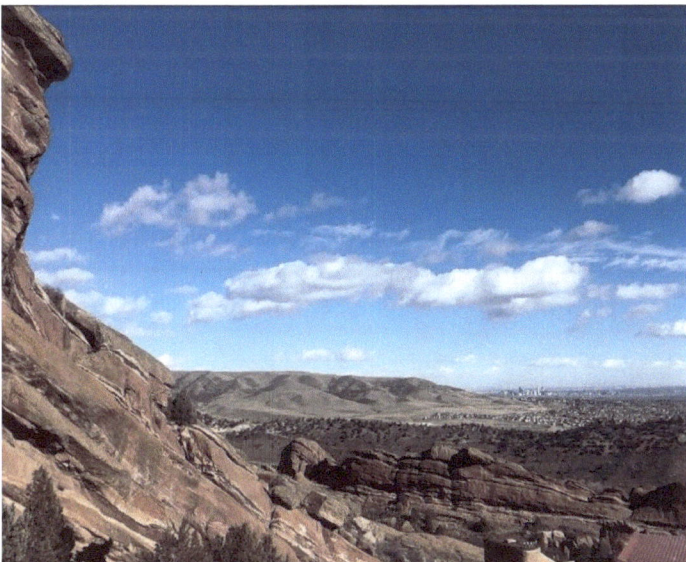

Chapter 16

BEAUTY CARE

People should be beautiful in every way—in their faces, in the way they dress, in their thoughts, and in their innermost selves.
– Anton Chekhov, Writer, 1860-1904

"Nothing makes a woman more beautiful than the belief that she is beautiful."
– Actress Sofia Loren

Every woman wants to look beautiful and orderly, presenting a fetching image both at work and at home. A neat look always makes a good impression; it strengthens a woman's sense of self-esteem and gives her more confidence in communicating. Style accents attractiveness and wearing fashionable clothes will make the wearer feel comfortable. Many women find men admire them if the woman portrays a pleasant smile, gentle behavior, and sincere feelings; although spiritual values are the foundation of true, never-ending beauty. These features are even more pronounced when a woman takes care of her appearance; for example, when she systematically takes care of her face, hands, and skin. By taking care of our external appearance, we also take care of our health.

When eating healthy food and taking daily exercises, even as simple as walking, we nourish both our body and skin. Consuming appropriate vitamins help as well. However, even more of these vitamins and minerals can be obtained by preparing facial masks. Masks are used to clean, nourish, and improve the blood circulation of the skin. They can revitalize the skin as they smooth out small wrinkles.

Having a beautiful skin does not require a lot of investment of time. The most important thing is a strict skin care routine. Cleaning, moisturizing, and nourishing should be performed both morning and evening. To wash away dead cells, nourish the pores, and leave your skin feeling smooth and refresh, avoid harsh chemicals. Instead, use natural moisturizers such as milk, honey, avocado, oatmeal, olive oil, banana, almonds, and aloe vera.

To refresh the skin, provide vitamins and minerals, and protect yourself against harmful environmental effects, an effective method is to spray yourself with mineral water, and then clean your face with milk and milk products. In the evening, wash your face with a chamomile tea decoction. This helps to soften the skin and unblock the pores.

If the skin is dry and sensitive or if wrinkles have already appeared, the best moisturizer product is milk which can moisturize the skin. Cleopatra, Queen of Ancient Egypt, took milk baths to preserve her beauty and youth. She often infused her milk bath with honey and herbs. These are both moisturizing and exfoliating. It leaves skin feeling silky and soft with a healthy glow. Do not use soap during these baths.

1. Royal milk bath: 2-4 cups of milk in a bath of warm water, soak for about 20 minutes. Brush and scrub the entire body. Rinse with warm water and pat dry with a soft towel.

2. Milk and honey bath:1-2 cups milk, ½ cup honey.

3. Dried flowers milk bath: 2 cups powdered milk, 1 tablespoon dried orange peels, 2 teaspoons dried lavender flowers, 2 teaspoons dried rosemary.

4. Essential oil milk bath: 1 cup powdered milk, ¼ baking soda, ¼ cup sea salt or Epsom salt, ¼ cup honey, ½ cup oats, dried or ground into powder, ¼ cup dried lavender flowers, 10-20 drops essential oil (optional).

When you are done, drain the tub and rinse yourself with water.

Another important hint: Try to protect your face from damage caused by cold temperatures and the sun. Wear a shade hat whenever you'll be out in the sun for more than fifteen minutes.

Facial Masks

Moisturizing and Hydrating Face Masks

1. Banana, coconut oil, sour cream. Mash ½ fully ripe banana in a mixing bowl. Add 2 teaspoons of coconut oil, 1 teaspoon of sour cream and mix thoroughly. Apply the puree to your clean and dry face and neck without touching the eye area. Leave this mask for 20 minutes and rinse with warm water, dry with soft towel.

2. Banana, honey. Mash one ripe banana in a mixing bowl. Add 2 tablespoons of raw honey and mix thoroughly. Stir 1 teaspoon of fresh-squeezed orange juice (optional). Massage the mask into your face. Leave it for 20 minutes. Rinse the mask off with warm water and dry with a clean, soft towel.

3. Banana, olive oil. If your facial skin is pale and delicate, pamper with bananas. Mash half the banana into a puree and add a few drops of cold-pressed olive oil. Leave for 10-15 minutes. Rinse with warm water and dry your face with a soft towel.

4. Aloe vera gel and cucumber. Cut ½ cucumber into slices. Place these slices in a blender or food processor and mix until watery. Add 2 tablespoons of aloe vera gel and

blend until smooth. Massage the paste evenly onto your face. After a half-hour, rinse off the mask with cool water and dry with a soft towel.

5. Vitamin E and avocado. Remove the pit and skin from half an avocado. Mash the avocado in a mixing bowl. Add 1 teaspoon of vitamin E oil. Mix well. Apply to the face and let it dry for 20 minutes. Wash with warm water and dry with a clean towel.

6. Strawberries, Greek yogurt and honey. Wash 3 medium size ripe strawberries, and puree with the blender. Spoon the puree into a bowl and add 2 teaspoons of Greek yogurt with 1 teaspoon of honey. Stir until the ingredients have a smooth consistency. Apply evenly to your face and leave this mask on for 10-15 minutes. If you have a dry skin type, 10 minutes is probably the best, whereas up to 15 minutes is better for an oily skin type.

7. Brewer's yeast, honey and milk. Mix well 1 tablespoon brewer's yeast and 1 tablespoon of honey. Stir in ¼ cup of warm milk. Mix until a smooth paste. Apply to your face and let it dry for 15 minutes. Wash with warm water, dry with a soft towel. A mask of yeast and warm milk revives and smooths the skin very quickly.

8. Papaya, honey, and milk. Remove the skin and take the seeds from 3 papaya slices and puree with the blender or food processor. Spoon the puree into a bowl with 1 teaspoon of honey and 2 teaspoons of milk. Stir well all ingredients together until evenly mixed. Apply the mixture to your face and rest for 20 minutes. Wash it off with warm water.

9. Avocado, egg yolk, and 1 tablespoon of honey. Mix well all ingredients, apply the mixture and leave it on for 10 minutes. Rinse with warm water. This mask will supply the skin with vitamins and smooth the face. After washing, you can use slices of cucumber or diluted lemon juice as a tonic, allowing the skin to tighten.

10. Honey, oatmeal and milk. Mix 3 tablespoons of dried oats with 1 tablespoon of whole milk until it develops into a paste. Drizzle in 1 tablespoon of honey. Apply the mixture to your face. Let the mask dry for 20 minutes and then wash it off with warm water. Dry with a soft towel.

Dry Skin

1. To soften dry skin, create a mask from one egg yolk with 3 tablespoons of sour cream. Smooth onto your face and let it rest for 15 minutes before rinsing with warm water. Use sour cream.

2. A mask of mashed egg yolk and sour cream softens dry skin. After 10-15 minutes, rinse first with warm water, then apply face cream. This anti-aging and antibacterial treatment feels non-greasy and absorbs easily.

3. For extra moisturizing, massage in 3-4 drops of olive oil twice a day. Here's another one: Blend 2 drops of almond oil, 1 tbsp of honey and 1 egg yolk together into a paste. Massage this into your face and leave for 20 minutes. Rinse with warm water and dry with a soft towel.

4. Mix a ¼ cup of yogurt, a ⅕ teaspoon of olive oil, and a ¼ of avocado together. Rub your face with this mixture and rinse with warm water after 15-20 minutes.
5. Honey. Put one teaspoon of bee honey in a glass with warm water, swirl until the honey melts and pour onto a cloth to wash your face. Let it stay for 10-15 minutes and rinse.
6. Bananas. Mash one banana and apply the mass to the face. Rinse with warm water after 10-15 minutes.
7. Aloe vera gel. Cut the aloe vera leaf diagonally and extract the gel. Apply some of this gel on your face and massage it in, so it is absorbed into the skin. Repeat this every night before going to bed.
8. Virgin coconut oil. Apply this oil on dry areas of your face and leave it on to get absorbed into the skin. This can be applied twice a day if needed.
9. Jojoba oil. This oil can be used as a face moisturizer as well as a body lotion.

Oily Skin

1. Mix a tablespoon of honey, a tablespoon of almond flour, and one egg yolk and apply the solution to your face and neck. Leave for 20 minutes, wash with warm water.
2. Cucumber cream cleans oily, unclean skin. Mash ½ a cucumber into a puree, add a few drops of raw organic and unfiltered Braggs apple cider vinegar. Leave for 10-15 minutes and wash it off with warm water, dry with soft towel. The resulting mixture cleans and tightens the skin. Never apply apple cider vinegar directly to the skin. It always has to be diluted with water 3:1.
3. Raw medium tomato: puree in the blender and apply to the face for 10-15 minutes before washing off.
4. Wheat flour. Take 4 tablespoons of whole-wheat flour, 3 tablespoons milk, 2 tablespoons raw honey. Bring milk to boil in a pan and then add rose water and honey. Remove the pan from the stove, slowly blend in wheat flour. Keep stirring till the paste thickens. Once cool, apply evenly on the face and neck. Wash off after 10-15 minutes.

Ready to use cream must be stored in a cool environment, otherwise it can expire very quickly. It is better to make one portion at a time (as it can be stored for a maximum of 8 days). Masks and deep cleansing remedies should be used immediately.

Be careful:

Use only fresh and clean substances and clean dishes for cosmetics.
Wash your hands well and clean your face before starting.
Always check that you are not allergic to one of the products by applying a small amount on a small area, for example, on the inside of the wrist.

Hair Care

1. Onion juice is a magical remedy for hair loss and baldness. Apply onion juice to problematic areas or the whole head and massage for at least 10 minutes. Cover your scalp with a cellophane bag and a cloth for 10 minutes. Repeat this procedure three times a week. The results will be simply stunning.
2. Rub the bald areas with freshly cut onions then apply small amounts of honey. Let it stay for 10 minutes and wash with warm water. Dry with a clean soft towel. Will help not only to prevent hair loss but also to restore some of the lost hair.
3. Boil a cup of water with rosemary. Use this solution to rinse your hair.
4. Eating nuts such as almonds and walnuts helps to grow hair, because they contain a high amount of magnesium.
5. Buy shampoos containing silicon dioxide, which promotes hair growth and helps to prevent hair loss.
6. Rosemary oil. Each night put two drops of this oil on your comb and gently comb it into your hair. Your hair will grow and be beautiful.
7. Salt spray for sexy beachy waves looking hair. Place 4 ounces (½ cup) of water in a spray bottle and add 1 tablespoon of kosher or sea salt to the water and shake. Mix a teaspoon of your favorite hair gel in the saltwater solution and shake it once again. After washing with shampoo and conditioner, spray onto wet hair to add texture and finger-comb only. Scrunch hair in your hands to help curls form, or just leave it be and let it air-dry naturally.
8. A balanced diet mix of vital nutrients such as proteins, vitamins, and minerals helps hair growth.

Hair Washing & Rinsing

Try not to wash your hair every day. Hair is damaged by frequent washing and drying with a hairdryer. Instead of using a hairdryer, let your hair dry naturally. Choose organic, natural shampoos that contain many different oils, such as coconut, argan, or macadamia. They will moisturize your hair without causing damage. The same rule applies to hair conditioners and balsams—try to use less aggressive chemicals.

Vinegar. Rinsing your hair with white vinegar or raw apple cider vinegar can give extra shine to your hair. It's better to use raw vinegar, rather than distilled, heated or clarified. Raw vinegar has much of the good bacteria, nutrients, and enzymes needed to improve hair texture.

To prepare a vinegar rinse, mix 2 cups of water with 4 tablespoons vinegar. After shampooing, pour the diluted vinegar onto the hair and wait 3-5 minutes before rinsing with cool water. Repeat one or twice a week to build up your hair and restore shine.

Although your hair may smell a little bit of vinegar for a short time, the smell will dissipate once your hair dries, leaving it soft and shiny. Note that rinsing with vinegar too often will make the hair dry and brittle.

Beer. Beer is a great product to achieve beautiful hair. Beer contains many minerals and vitamins that give the hair firmness, shine, and extra strength. It's particularly effective on thin or delicate hair. The malt and hops in a beer are rich in protein that help repair damaged hair and revive volume. As well, the sucrose and maltose sugars in beer create shine. If your hair is looking a little dull or flat, a bottle of beer might be the answer.

1. Before washing your hair, you'll need to decarbonate the beer. Pour the beer into a bowl and let it sit overnight or throughout the day. Beer becomes flat by releasing its carbon dioxide.

2. Shampoo with your normal shampoo, but don't use conditioner.

3. Pour the beer into your hair and lather your scalp. Massage for 1 minute and let it sit for 3-4 minutes. Rinse lightly with cool water. If preferred, you can skip the rinse for better effect. Dry with a soft towel. The beer odor will dissipate in a few minutes. It may take several washes before you feel and see results. Beer treatment should be limited to once or twice a week; rinsing with beer too often will make the hair dry.

Beer is also beneficial for your skin, helping to control oily skin.

Hair Mask

To maintain healthy and glossy hair, before every wash mix an egg yolk with a tablespoon of castor oil (or other oils) and rub your hair from the root to the ends. Hold this mask for about 10 minutes and rinse thoroughly.

Make Hands Soft and Beautiful

1. Boil two potatoes with their skins left on and add a few teaspoons of milk, kefir, or sour cream. Mix everything thoroughly and apply the paste to your hands. After 10-30 min., rinse first with warm water and then again with cold water. Apply hand cream to wet hands.

2. Mix ½ teaspoon of olive oil to 1 teaspoon of sugar and rub this mixture into your palms, covering the skin. Gently rinse with water.

3. Mix 1 tablespoon each of glycerin and rosewater, add a squeeze of lemon juice, stir well and rub it into your hands. Dry with a soft towel. Apply twice a day.

4. Soak hands in egg yolk. Put the egg yolk into a small bowl, add 1 teaspoon of honey, ½ teaspoon of almond oil. Stir well. Leave mixture for 10 minutes, gently rinse and dry.

5. Lemon and sugar. Take ½ slice of fresh lemon and sprinkle a little sugar on the moist fruit. Squeeze into your hand until the sugar seems completely gone.

6. Make a hand scrub with coconut oil. Put 1 tablespoon coconut oil into a small bowl, add 2 tablespoons honey and mix well. In a second bowl mix ¼ cup sea salt with ¼ cup sugar, add 1 tablespoon lemon juice to the dry mixture until it has the consistency of slightly damp sand. Combine the salt mixture with the oil and honey mixture and stir well. Rub into your hands. Rinse with warm water and gently dry with a soft towel. Store excess scrub in a glass jar with a lid. Apply 1-2 times a week.

Make Your Hands Look Younger

1. Wear gloves when you're washing dishes or working in a garden.
2. Moisturize. I recommend treatments like shea butter, olive oil, vitamin E and macadamia oil. Apply these to slightly damp skin, which helps them absorb better.
3. Wear sunscreen.
4. Exfoliate, exfoliate. Use a gentle exfoliator- nothing too abrasive, because it can scratch the skin surface. Try using a teaspoon of sugar combined with coconut oil, or olive oil and sugar.

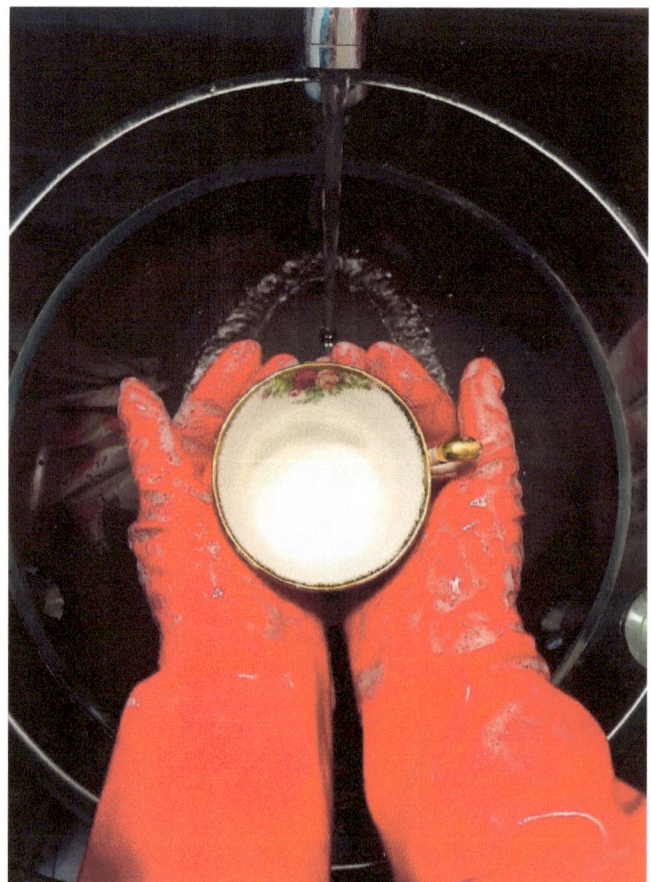

Chapter 17

SILENT KILLERS AT HOME

The definition of genius is taking the complex and making it simple. – Albert Einstein, 1879-1955, Physicist and Nobel Laureate.

British and American doctors and researchers warn of the following silent killers in your home:

1. Scented candles and air fresheners release toxic chemicals that can cause a variety of health problems including cancer, asthma, lung, cardiovascular disease, diabetes, obesity, and dementia. Some studies found they adversely affect the development of the fetus and the male genitalia, which may cause birth defects and reproductive problems. Even the scent of the lemon or pine used in scented candles and home air fresheners can release toxic fumes. In these products, the pleasant scent of lemon is made up of limonene. When limonene mixes with other airborne contaminants, it can transform into formaldehyde, increasing the risk of throat and nasal cancer. Limonene is not the only harmful chemical in scented candles. Its composition is usually made up of chemical products that can produce benzene, lead, and other chemicals. Scented candles are more dangerous than ordinary candles as they emit more chemical particles.

2. Shampoo and shower gel. We use shower gel or shampoo every time we take a shower. However, such cleansers can be harmful to your health, especially if they contain anti-inflammatory substances, sodium lauryl sulfate (SLS), or triclosan, which, according to the American College of Toxicology, can cause skin irritation, even in small quantities. Higher concentrations of these substances can lead to severe skin diseases. These aforementioned chemicals are used for motor and garage floor washing, but they are also added to shampoos, soaps, and other cosmetic products. You can find better alternatives to shampoo and body scrubs in natural and biocosmetic stores or online. We recommend trying a few of these brands; "A Soap for Goodness Sake," "Ethical," and "Dr. Woods Products."

3. Dishwashing detergent. No matter how thoroughly you rinse the dishes, if you wash them with a dish detergent, toxic particles are still left on your plates, cups, glasses, and cutlery, and they inevitably fall into your mouth. In addition, like most commercial shampoos, many dishwasher detergents contain harmful substances such as sodium lauryl sulfate (SLS) and triclosan, not to mention the popular "scented" dishwashing detergents. Thus, we recommend choosing dishwasher

detergents manufactured by "Better Life," Imus GTC," "Attitude," and "Whole Foods Market."

After washing dishes in a dishwashing machine, pour a glass of white vinegar into the dishwasher and rinse the dishes that have already been washed. This will disinfect the dishes and remove the remaining chemicals that are attached to the walls of the dishes.

4. Dry cleaners. Be aware that clothes returning from the dry cleaners will still have dangerous chemicals in them. All clothes from a dry cleaners should be well ventilated outside before wearing.

5. Antibacterial soap. Do not use antibacterial soap. Follow the classic method of hot water and natural soap without any harmful chemicals. While using antibacterial soap, good bacteria are also removed; in turn, this weakens our immunity in the long run. This soap also dries the skin, making it much easier for viruses to enter our body. The antibacterial products have been blamed for the increase in superbugs in our environment.

WAYS TO REDUCE INDOOR AIR POLLUTION

1. Buy plants. Indoor plants clean air. They inhale carbon dioxide and breathe oxygen through their leaves. Plants cleanse the air and help to clean the indoor air due to their natural ability to absorb toxins through leaves and roots and turn them into nutrients.
Dr. Wolverton recommends bamboo palm (Chamaedorea seifrizii), aglaonema (Aglaonema modestum), ivy (Hedera helix), Barberton daisy (Gerbera jamesonii), and aloe vera (Aloe vera barbadensis). The aloe plant is especially beneficial when situated in the bedroom.
2. Use environmentally friendly cleaning agents. How do you recognize if a cleaning agent is harmful? Avoid products with product packaging warnings like: "this product is unsafe for the environment."
3. Buy "green" products. Some low-emission carpets, paints, and building materials are marked with special labels indicating that they produce the least amount of chemicals. Such labeling can be varied. For example, low emission carpets are labeled "Green Label" and "Green Label plus."
4. Do not keep windows closed—open them and inhale fresh air into your living space.

15 toxic household products you should stop buying.

1. Laundry products. Some brands, such as Ajax, Dynamo, and Fab Ultra contain formaldehyde, which can cause asthma and allergies. Their partners-in-crime, scented dryer sheets, are no better and should be avoided.

2. Nonstick cookware. Contains trace amounts of perfluorooctanoic acid. This chemical has been proven to cause cancer in lab animals. Nonstick surfaces may chip off into your food and enter your body. To avoid this, only use cast iron or stainless steel pans and invest in some natural cooking sprays or oils.

3. Air fresheners. These products have some nasty side effects, Formaldehyde and phenol are common ingredients.

4. Toilet bowl cleaners. Sulfates and bleach are commonly found in toilet bowl cleaners. Therefore, as you bend down to scrub the toilet, you are probably breathing in a toxic chlorine gas that is extremely dangerous to your respiratory and circulatory systems.

5. Plastic food containers. They release chemicals into food wrap and containers, including a hormone similar to estrogen into the substances it stores. One study even claims that BPA-free content may be leaking chemicals into food and drink.

6. Oven cleaners. Poisonous ingredients that can lead to difficulty breathing, swelling of the throat, vision loss, abdominal pain, and vomiting are found in many of these types of products.

7. Make up. Contains propylene glycol methylparaben and propylparaben. Lipstick and mascara may also contain these ingredients. Pay extra for high-end products that don't contain these chemicals.

8. Furniture polish. Contains hydrocarbons which have toxic vapors.

9. Window cleaners. High content of the toxic isopropyl alcohol, also known by its more common name, rubbing alcohol. The fumes can cause headache, vomiting, and dizziness.

10. Fertilizer. Nitrates are a form of nitrogen that cause allergic reactions, skin irritation, and poisonous if ingested.

11. Drain cleaners. Drain cleaners are among the most dangerous of all cleaning products. Most contain corrosive ingredients such as sodium hydroxide and sodium hypochlorite (bleach). Chemical drain cleaners are dangerous when they come into contact with any part of the body, burning the skin and ruining the eyes. Damage to the esophagus if drunk can be fatal.

12. Insect repellents. DEET or diethyltoluamide, a strong and dangerous pesticide, is the most common active ingredient in insect repellents. DEET has been implicated as causing seizures and brain malfunction, cancer, pet toxicity, and a severe environmental impact.

13. Mildew removers. This product contains sodium hypochloride, which could cause respiratory issues or eye and skin irritation if you don't use it in a well-ventilated area.

14. Scented lotions. These products typically found in insecticides and wood finishes, contain phthalates, carcinogenic parabens, and BHA - butylated hydroxyanisole that disrupt your endocrine system. Although they may smell like strawberries and cream, they are toxic chemicals.

15. Mothballs. Mothballs contain either naphthalene or paradichlorobenze as active ingredients. The Department of Health and Human Services (DHHS) concluded that naphthalene is reasonably anticipated to be a human carcinogen which destroys red blood cells causing hemolytic anemia. Symptoms of exposure to chemicals include headache, nausea, dizziness, and difficulty breathing.

Weaknesses of Ticks and Mosquitoes

If you spend a lot of time in nature in the summer, it is important to take care of the safety of our beloved pets. Here are some helpful tips:

Tea tree oil. Mosquitoes and ticks do not like the tea tree oil.

Mix 10 drops of essential tea tree oil with 50 ml of water and pour into a spray vial. Shake well and spray over open areas of the body and clothes.

Dogs are allergic to tree oil.

Vinegar. Vinegar acts as a natural repellent. Add 1 part vinegar to 1 part water. Add 10 drops of essential eucalyptus or peppermint oil to the spray vial. Sprinkle this mixture every few hours.

Garlic. Ticks cannot stand the scent of garlic. Add to your own menu while you are on holiday, or rub open body areas with garlic juice.

Neem oil: Melia azadirachta (Indian lilac). This oil is very commonly used in ayurvedic medicine and also protects against ticks. Mix 5-10 drops with a cup of water and rub on open areas of the body.

Citrus fruits. Like garlic, ticks cannot tolerate the scent of citrus fruits. The best fruit to use is a green or yellow lemon because their scent is the best. Boil 2 sliced fruits in 2 cups of water for 1 hour, filter, and pour into a bottle. All the family can use it and it also can be used for pets and the lawn.

For animals. Ticks often come home crawling in our pets' fur. They are particularly fond of attaching themselves to dogs and cats while in the grass. Essential oil mixtures can also help in such cases. Some pets are often allergic to these products and can only tolerate a very small amount of them. The best way is to eradicate the location of the ticks that are in the fur by rubbing with a thick Vaseline layer. The ticks will not be able to breathe and will fall out within a few days.

Once tick season is on the increase, always check your body carefully to get rid of this unpleasant blood parasite in time. Ticks not only have an unpleasant appearance, but they also carry dangerous diseases that have irreversible consequences when they embed themselves in the skin. It takes 24 hours for a tick to pass an infection to a human, so early removal can prevent transmission.

Natural, homemade safety measures can be very useful for you. Just make sure you are not allergic to any ingredient and avoid getting the product into the nose, eyes, or mouth.

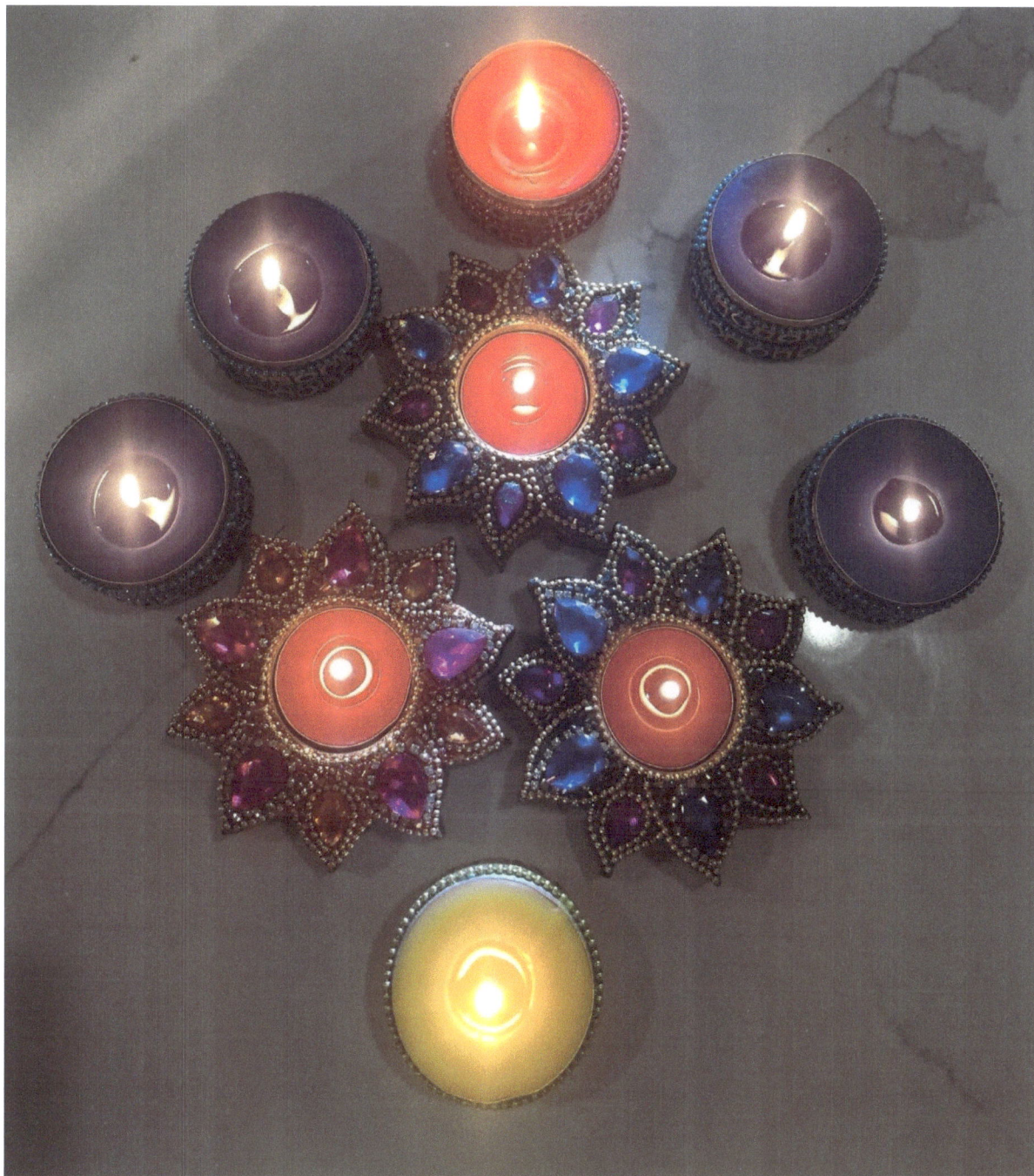

Chapter 18

HOUSEHOLD USES OF NATURAL PRODUCTS

"Don't call the world dirty because you forget to clean your glasses".
— Aaron Hill, professional baseball third baseman.

Baking Soda (Sodium Bicarbonate)

Sodium Bicarbonate is a natural mineral found in large quantities throughout the world, including Searles Lake, California, the Piceance Basin of the Green River Formation in Colorado, and in Botswana, Kenya, Uganda, Turkey, and Mexico. It comes out of the ground in the form of minerals nahcolite and natron, which are refined into soda ash (calcium carbonate), then turned into baking soda (sodium bicarbonate). When taking care of ecological life and clean nature, use simple baking soda which is easy to break down and does not harm the soil, plants, or animals. By choosing natural baking soda instead of chemicals, detergents, or bleaches, we can clean while protecting nature and decrease allergies, asthma, and cancer. Baking soda is an ideal substitute for many personal hygiene products that are full of toxic substances, such as aluminum in deodorants and parabens in creams.

Personal Hygiene

1. Eliminate bad mouth odors. Rinse your mouth with a soda solution (a teaspoon of soda per glass of warm water).
2. Soak dental prostheses. Dissolve 2 teaspoons of soda in a glass of water and soak dental prostheses in the glass. The soda will release the remaining food residues and eliminate odors.
3. Scrub face and body. Make a paste comprising 3 parts soda and 1 part water. With gentle circular motions, rub face and body skin to remove the dry skin layer. Rinse well with water.
4. Deodorant. A commonly used personal hygiene product that you are most likely to use every morning or several times a day is a deodorant. Deodorants include a range of toxins, including breast cancer parabens, aluminum, and triclosan, which can potentially cause Alzheimer's disease. To protect the bloodstream and the lymphatic system from these harmful toxins, an effective alternative is the natural mineral deodorant baking soda. After your shower, rub the damp underarms with soda and let them dry. There will be no sweaty smell and no chemical reactions. As an adjunct, consider adding cornstarch which absorbs wetness and odor. Mix ½ soda with ½ cornstarch

Homemade Deodorant Recipe

In a pot add 1 tablespoon of coconut oil, 1 tablespoon of soda, and 1 tablespoon of cornstarch. Cook the coconut oil on a low heat until the oil dissolves. Slowly pour the soda and starch out and shake well. The mass must be very thick. If you have an old deodorant dish, pour the resulting mixture into it and store in the refrigerator.

5. Dry Shampoo. For light hair. ¼ cup corn starch, ¼ cup baking soda, 1 tsp cinnamon, 3-5 drops essential oil (optional).
For dark hair. ¼ corn starch, ¼ cup baking soda, ¼ cup cocoa powder or ¼ cup cinnamon, 3-5 drops essential oil (optional).
Put dry ingredients in a mixing bowl, add essential oil and blend all the ingredients well. Transfer this into a jar, salt shaker, empty spice jar, or an empty Parmesan cheese container to store dry shampoo. This will give you an easy way to sprinkle it on your hair.
6. To suppress itching after an insect bite. Make a paste with soda and water and apply to infected site. To relieve itching, rub the soda on wet skin.
7. Make hair more beautiful. Not only is vinegar an excellent remedy for hair, but soda is also appropriate. Take a pinch of soda, add a shampoo, and wash head as usual. Soda will remove the remains of hair styling products and so make it easier to style.
8. Make a soda bath. Add ½ cup of soda to a bathtub. Stay in the bath for 20-25 minutes. You can also mix soda with Epsom or sea salts. Such a bath relaxes the body, eliminates the negative energy accumulated from the body during the day, and speeds up blood circulation. Soda neutralizes acid from the skin and removes grease and sweat, leaving the skin feeling gentle to the touch.
Noteworthy: The Epsom salt and soda in a bath is a miraculous remedy. Even after bathing, it continues its work. Therefore, do not take a shower after this kind of bath. After getting out of the bath, dry gently, don a bathrobe, and drink hot tea.
9. Soften feet skin. Dissolve 3 tablespoons of soda in a warm water bath and soak your feet. Your feet will remain soft and gentle and the sweat scent will disappear.
10. Clean hair brushes and combs. Your hair will not shine if you comb it with a dirty or greasy comb. Instead, before brushing, first soak the comb in a warm soda solution (1 teaspoon soda in a glass of water), rinse, and dry.

Cleaning

1. Homemade Mild Surface Cleaner. To make a safe and effective tool to clean baths, sinks, and tiles, place soda on a damp sponge and scrub. Be sure to rinse and dry thoroughly with water. Soda dissolves fat, so it can be used instead of dishwashing detergent.

Homemade dishwasher detergent: Add about two-three drops of regular dish soap to your dishwasher's detergent cup. Fill the cup 2/3 with baking soda. Add salt until the cup is nearly full.

2. Refresh sponge and washcloths. Soak stinky sponges in a strong soda solution (4 tablespoons in half a liter of warm water). Wash with clean water.

3. Clean the microwave. You can clean the microwave with baking soda on a damp sponge—it will not smell of chemicals.

4. Scrub silver dishes. Make a paste comprising 3 parts soda and 1 part water. Scrub and rinse thoroughly with water.

5. Clean the oven. Sprinkle a large amount of soda on the bottom of the oven. Sprinkle with water to moisten the soda and leave overnight. Scrub in the morning, wipe the rest of the soda away, and rinse the oven with water.

6. Wash the floor. Dissolve ½ cup of soda in a bucket of warm water and wash an unwaxed, tiled, or cement floor. Rinse with clean water. The floor will shine like new.

7. Clean the furniture. Gently rub furniture and walls with a damp sponge with soda. Wipe with a dry clean cloth.

8. Clean bathroom curtains. Clean the curtains and revive their scent by brushing with soda on a damp sponge or brush. Rinse with water and dry.

9. Refresh smells of sport bags. Sprinkle your sport bags with soda, leave for some time, and then beat the dust out.

10. Remove stains from grease and oil. If you notice fat stains on garage floors or patio paving, rub them with soda, leave for some time, and rinse them with a water stream.

11. Wash cars. Use the soda for washing lights, chrome fittings, windows, tires, and vinyl seats without worrying about scratches. Add a ¼ cup of soda to a liter of warm water.

12. Clean your windows perfectly. Clean with a damp cloth and soda, and then rinse with another cloth soaked in hot water.

13. Bathroom, toilet, shower wall. You can easily clean these areas with a paste made of 1 part of soda and ½ part vinegar. This paste not only scrubs but also removes soap and molds.

14. Clean and deodorize the dishwasher. Sprinkle soda in the dishwasher to eliminate odor. When the washing mode is switched on, the soda will improve the effect of the detergent.

15. Eliminate odors of carpets and furniture upholstery. Sprinkle a large amount of soda directly onto the carpet or furniture. Leave overnight or even longer, then wipe and vacuum with a vacuum cleaner. At the same time, you will deodorize the vacuum cleaner.

Odor Removal

1. Refresh the odor in the closets. Put an open jar of soda on the shelf of the closet.

2. Removing refrigerator odors. Simply leave an uncovered jar with soda in the fridge rack.

3. Remove the odor from cutting boards. Sprinkle soda on the cutting board, scrub and rinse.

4. Remove the odor of the trash can. Sprinkle soda on the bottom of the tank. Periodically wash the tank with soda solution.

5. Deodorize drainage pipelines. In order to avoid bad smells emanating from the sink, add ½ cup of soda to the drainage hole and pour warm water down it. If the sink is clogged, pour ½ a cup of soda and ½ a cup of white vinegar. When the bubbles disappear, rinse with hot water.

6. Baking soda absorbs odors. You will need a cup of baking soda for a large dog or half a cup for a small dog. Sprinkle baking soda onto your dog's coat (avoid the face) and let it sit for a few minutes to absorb odor. Brush the baking soda and use a hand towel in a drying motion to remove any excess.

7. If your dog or cat gets wet in the rain and the fur spreads an unpleasant odor, wipe the fur with soda. The odor will disappear and the fur will dry faster.

Cooking

1. You can use baking soda as a replacement for baking powder in most recipes. By releasing carbon dioxide, the soda expands the dough, creating a fluffy product. The famous Russian blini uses kefir and baking soda as dough rising agents, often eaten with sour cream.

2. Washing fruits and vegetables. Soda is the best and most harmless tool to wash away all dirt from fruit and vegetables. Soak them in a concentrated soda solution after taking from the store. One handful of soda for one liter of water. It dissolves chemicals perfectly. Rinse with clean water after 15-20 minutes. The synthetics will disappear, and the natural fruit will remain.

Other Tips

1. An indispensable tool for traveling and getting around. If you are going to spend time in nature, take some soda, which will be needed as a dishwasher, deodorant, toothpaste, or even as a fire extinguisher.

2. Baking soda is the first means of extinguishing a small fire of burning fats. Simply squeeze the soda on the fire to extinguish it.

3. If the stairs are covered with ice in winter, sprinkle them with soda.

4. If you smoke, fill the ashtray with soda. This will eliminate the odors of tobacco smoke.

5. You will extend the life of flowers by adding 1 teaspoon of sugar with 1 teaspoon of soda to the vase.

Household Uses for Vinegar

Vinegar is not only used for salad dressings; its liquid is also beneficial to our household.
1. Vinegar is an irreplaceable measure along with a washing machine. It bleaches, gives tissues a more distinct color, and it removes unpleasant odors. Vinegar can be used instead of an industrial laundry softener. Add half a glass of vinegar to the rinse section in the washing machine and vinegar will help to remove the detergent residues from the tissues. Clothes will remain softer. It is also great for rinsing clothes, as it minimizes the impact on allergy sufferers, as better rinsed clothes will not irritate the skin.
2. When washing white tissues, vinegar will act as a natural bleach. To restore the brightness of white cotton clothes, pour a glass of vinegar into a hot bath and leave the clothes in it overnight. Then, wash them according to the instructions on the label. Before washing shirts, it is recommended to pour vinegar on the sweatiest places, such as the armpits and the collar area. Vinegar will help you get rid of the unpleasant smell and prevent the material from tarnishing.
3. To clean the burn marks from an iron, scrub the area with a warm mixture of edible salt and vinegar. Then wipe it off with a damp cloth soaked in strong vinegar.
4. When the kitchen sink drainage is clogged, vinegar will help to break up the clog and at the same time eliminate the unpleasant smells that occasionally emerge from those tubes. Add ½ a cup of baking soda and 1 cup of vinegar to the drain pipe. The fluid will start bubbling from the tube. When the liquid stops bubbling, rinse with hot tap water followed by cold water. The drainage pipe will be clean and free of clogs.
5. Ink stains on tablecloths, shirts, etc. can be removed by pouring a little vinegar (white only) on a soft cloth or sponge and soak the spotty area. Repeat until the ink disappears.
6. Mold stains in the bathroom or elsewhere (e.g. in a refrigerator) can be cleaned with vinegar. If there are many stains, use undiluted vinegar. If there are only slight stains, use diluted vinegar with cold water. Vinegar will not be harmful to any surface and it is not toxic for breathing, unlike other chemicals for mold cleaning.
7. If glue is too dry, add a few drops of vinegar, store it for at least 12 hours overnight, then stir. The glue will be liquid again.
8. The glass of windows and mirrors will be clean and shine beautifully after washing with an equal parts of water and vinegar solution.
9. After washing crystalline vases, rinse with an equal parts of water and vinegar solution. The vases will shine.
10. Cut flowers in the vase will last longer in water by adding 2 tablespoons of vinegar and 2 teaspoons of sugar.

11. In a dishwasher machine, white vinegar can be a great rinse aid, giving a glossy sheen to glasses, plates, and dishes. White vinegar is a common rinse aid for detergents. Mild acid will rinse off cleaning solution such as dishwasher detergent. The surfactants in dishwasher soap will leave a white detergent residue on dishes if not thoroughly rinsed away. Fill the rinse agent dispenser with the vinegar and close the lid, or twist the cap shut. Remove all metal or silverware as vinegar may damage them. If your dishwasher does not have a rinse aid dispenser, fill a glass with 2 cups of vinegar. Place the cup in the bottom rack of the dishwasher and run the dishwasher as normal. Remove all metal or silverware.

If you want to clear away odors from your dishwasher, pour a cup of vinegar into an empty dishwasher machine and wash with a short wash cycle.

12. To heal nail fungus, soak them in a warm bath of vinegar (dilute the water at a ratio of 1:5) for 15-20 minutes daily for a few days.

Coca-Cola: Not Just for the Stomach

The famous beverage Coca-Cola is not only a drink; it is also good for your household.

1. Polish the toilet. Pour a bottle's worth of Coca-Cola into the toilet and leave it for 1 hour, then clean with a brush and flush. The toilet will gloss again.

2. The same can be done with burnt pots.

3. Remove stains from clothing. Mix with a laundry detergent in equal parts and pour it into the washing machine. Coca-Cola will not only remove blood, paint, or fat stains, but it will also eliminate the odor of unpleasant clothing.

4. Coca-Cola cleans old coins perfectly. Simply place the coins in a bowl of Coca-Cola. After a while, remove the coins and wipe with a water-soaked cloth so that they do not stick.

5. Clean rust. If you want to remove rust from iron tools, soak them in a full bowl of Coca-Cola. You can unscrew rusty screws with Coca-Cola. Pour this beverage over your old screws and wait a few minutes before rinsing.

6. Reduce the pain of insect bites. If you have a mosquito or bee bite on your holiday, or if stung by a jellyfish while swimming in the sea, pour some Coca-Cola on the affected site and the pain will pass away in a few seconds.

7. Get rid of insects. When relaxing in nature, flying insects rarely leave humans in peace. To keep them at bay, open some Coca-Cola cans or pour Coca-Cola in glasses. The odor of Coca-Cola will attract all the insects. Instead of Coca-Cola, Pepsi Cola can also be used.

Hydrogen peroxide

Hydrogen peroxide is a colorless liquid compound of hydrogen and oxygen. Its chemical formula is H2O2. It is a mild antiseptic for cuts, scrapes and burns, and a very strong oxidizing and bleaching agent. Viscous when pure, hydrogen peroxide can be mixed with water in any proportion. Unstable, it rapidly decomposes into water.

Some Common Uses of Hydrogen Peroxide

1. It disinfects small scratches and cuts.
2. Soak toothbrushes with hydrogen peroxide to disinfect them.
3. Clean the surfaces of the kitchen and cutting boards with hydrogen peroxide. Spray, let it bubble, and rinse thoroughly with water. It is particularly important after slicing meat or fish as peroxide will kill microbes.
4. Clean the toilet. Pour a cup of peroxide into the toilet bowl and let it soak for about 20 minutes before scrubbing.
5. Peroxide bleaches stains from white linen. Just sprinkle the stain with the peroxide before washing or add peroxide directly to the washing machine along with the detergent. Be careful: Before spraying on the stain, try the peroxide on a small remote part of the shirt to be sure it won't damage the color.
6. Clean the floor. In a bucket of water, add a cup of peroxide and wash as usual. There will be no need to wash again. The solution is very clean and does not harm any type of floor.
7. Bleach the curtains. Fill a sink full of water, add 1-2 glasses of peroxide, and soak the curtains for about an hour. Following this, rinse and dry.
8. Peroxide helps to treat nail and foot fungus. When going to bed, spray your feet and fingers with water-dissolved peroxide in equal parts. Or soak your feet in such a solution.

Useful liquid

Chlorine (bleach) is one of the most useful liquids when we want to remove stains from laundry or dishes, or to disinfect. It smells unpleasant and its steam makes the eyes smart. Despite being poisonous, it is an irreplaceable weapon against molds, bacteria, and various pests. However, you should take care to not mix chlorine with other chemicals such as ammonia due to the appearance of dangerous gases. When using chlorine, it is advisable to protect your hands with rubber gloves and wear protective goggles and a face mask.

1. If you add 1 teaspoon to the dishwasher, the glasses and other vessels will be very clean and shine brightly.
2. When you add a little chlorine to a washing machine, the laundry will be clean and stains will disappear.

3. Cut flowers will blossom longer in the vase if you add a few drops of chlorine water. Also, the water will not have a smell and the vase will remain clean.

4. If grass starts to grow on the cement path near the entry of a house, spray undiluted chlorine cleaner on the grass. The grass will not only disappear, but others will not grow in that area. Spraying chlorine on flowers destroys them, so spraying requires care.

5. Pour a little chlorine on the flowing fountain to destroy the mosquito eggs. Chlorine will suspend the growth of moorings in stagnant water.

6. Leave used flower-pots to soak in a chlorine solution (4 parts water, 1 part chlorine): the flower-pots will be clean, free from contamination, and suitable for new plants.

Salt

As salt is not expensive, it can not only be used for food but also for cleaning and other things.

1. If your enamel pot is burnt, add water, a couple of tablespoons of salt, and leave overnight. In the morning, boil the water in the pot, pour it out, and the pot will be cleaned.

2. Sprinkle salt on the tablecloth with fruit and berry juice stains. The stains will be washed away.

3. Carpet runners are easy to clean with a sponge soaked in a salt solution.

4. If you cannot light a fire in the fireplace, add a little salt, causing the fire to blaze almost immediately.

5. If your hands have the odor of onions or fish, the odor will disappear after washing them in salted water.

6. To boil potatoes with uncracked peels, add half a teaspoon of salt to the water.

7. To keep the salt from getting moist in the kitchen, throw a few rice grains into the salt cellar.

8. If you wipe car windows with salted water (inside and outside), they will not freeze.

9. If artificial flowers are dusty or otherwise greased, put the blossoms in a paper bag, add salt, close, and shake well. The salt will remove dust and dirt.

10. If fat has baked onto the oven, pour a layer of salt on the stained area. Once the fat is absorbed in the salt, rinse the oven with a damp sponge.

11. To remove stains from glass or other dishes, soak a damp sponge or cloth with salt and rub the stained area, then rinse and dry it: the salt will not scratch the glass unlike cleaning powder.

How to Clean Anything

1. The acidity of lemon juice removes dirt and rust. Adding a little salt to the juice makes if more effective for cleaning, especially for removing rust.

2. Plastic (as well as wooden) cutting boards for meat or other products should be thoroughly cleaned using the following method: cut a lemon in half, squeeze the juice onto the plate, keep it for 20 minutes, and then wash and dry.

3. Plastic containers used in microwaves or to store food in a refrigerator sometimes turn the color of the food they contain (e.g., tomato juice). Rub the stained areas with lemon juice until they have lost their stain, then rinse as usual.

4. If the water runs slowly from the tap or the shower due to the accumulation of sediment, rub lemon juice over the spout and leave overnight. The acid will eliminate sediment.

Oil: it is usually used for food preparation, especially when cooking or baking, but it can also be a cleanser.

1. Cast-iron pans are well cleaned by making a paste of oil and a spoonful of salt. Apply this paste to the inside of the pan, rinse it with hot water, and drain it. If you have not used cast-iron pans for a long time, the inside of the pans can develop a rust layer. To prevent this from happening, rinse the frying pan, dry, and then apply a thin layer of oil.

2. To remove paint from your hands, try rubbing them with oil, then wash them with soap and water.

3. To remove scratches from either dirty or dust-free leather shoes, pour a few drops of oil and wax them with a soft cloth.

4. In order for wicker furniture (usually used outdoors in the summer) to not dry or crumble, rub it with warmed oil (the oil will be more liquid and it is easier to cover the surface of the furniture), then wipe it with a soft cloth.

5. Wooden furniture is cleaned beautifully with a mixture of oil and lemon juice. Simply add 2 tablespoons of oil, the juice of one lemon, and mix well. This ointment can be stored in the refrigerator for a long period of time.

Glossary

Abscesses: A collection of pus that has built up within the tissue of the body.

Acesulfame-potassium: Also known as acesulfame K or ACEK is a calorie-free sugar substitute.

AIDS: Human immunodeficiency virus infection and acquired immune deficiency syndrome.

Allergen: Any antigen that causes allergy in a hypersensitive person.

Allergy: Allergic diseases, are a number of conditions caused by hypersensitivity of the immune system to typically harmless substances in the environment.

Alzheimer: Chronic neurogenerative disease that usually starts and worsens over time. A progressive form of dementia.

Ancient: Refer to anything considered "very old".

Anesthetizing: Administer an anesthetic to a person or animal, especially so as to induce a loss of sensation or consciousness.

Antibacterial: Anything that destroys bacteria or suppresses their growth.

Antibiotics: A type of antimicrobial substance active against bacteria used to fight bacterial infections.

Antidepressant: Medications that can help relieve symptoms of depression, social anxiety, mild chronic depression, as well as other condition.

Anthrax: An infection caused by bacterium Bacillus anthracis.

Antioxidants: Are found in many foods, including fruits and vegetables. They are also available as dietary supplements.

Antiseptic: Is a substance that stops or slows down the growth of microorganism.

Aphrodisiac: A food, drink or drug that stimulates sexual desire. A thing that causes excitement.

Aromatherapy: Uses plant materials and romantic plant oils, including essential oils other aroma compounds for improving psychological or physical well-being.

Arteriosclerosis: The thickening and hardening of the walls of the arteries, occurring typically in old age.

Asclepius: In ancient Greek mythology, a god of medicine and healing.

Atherosclerosis: Is a disease in which the inside of an artery narrows due to the build up of plaque.

Athlete's foot: (tinea pedis) Is a fungal infection that usually begins between the toes. It commonly occurs in people whose feet have become sweaty and not cleaned and dried properly. It's a scaly rash that usually causes itching, stinging, and burning.

Avicenna:(Ibn Sina). Persian polymath who is regarded as one of the most significant physicians of the Islamic Golden Age.

Ayran.: Is a cold savory yogurt based beverage that is mixed with salt.

Ayurvedic medicine: As practiced in India, is one of the oldest system of medicine in the world.

Baking soda: is a natural mineral (Sodium Bicarbonate).

Beta-carotene: Is an antioxidant that converts to vitamin A and plays a very important role in healing.

Beta-glucans: Comprise a group of B-D-glucose polysaccharides naturally occurring in the all walls of cereals, bacteria, and fungi with significant physiochemical properties dependent on source.

Bio energy: Renewable energy produced by living organisms.

Blood platelets: A structure in blood relating to the arrest of bleeding.

Botulism: Is a rare potentially fatal illness caused by a toxin produced by the bacterium Clostridium botulinum.

Calluses: Is an area of thickened skin that forms as a response to repeated friction, pressure or other irritation.

Cannabis: (Cannabis sativa). Also known as Marijuana among other names, is a psychoactive drug from the Cannabis plant.

Cancer: A malignant tumor.

Cardiac: Relating to the heart.

Carotenoids: Soluble pigments.

Cartilage: Firm, whitish, flexible connective tissue found in various forms.

Cellulite: Accumulation of toxins due to an excess of fat in the tissue.

Chlorophyll: A green pigment, present in all green plants.

Cholesterol: Fat-like material in blood and most tissues.

Cirrhosis: Is a late stage of scarring of the liver caused by many forms of liver disease and conditions, typically alcoholism.

Collagen: Is the main structural protein in the extracellular space in the various connective tissues in animal bodies.

Colic: Severe, often fluctuating pain in the abdomen caused by intestinal gas or obstruction in the intestines and suffered especially by babies.

Dementia: A chronic or persistent disorder of the mental processes caused by brain disease or injury.

Depilation: Is the deliberate removal of the body hair.

Depressant: Reduces nervous or functional activity.

Dermatitis: (Also known as eczema). Inflammation of the skin typically causing a pink or red itchy rash.

Deterioration: The process of becoming progressively worse.

Diabetes: Any disorder of the metabolism causing excessive thirst and the production of large volumes of urine. Most commonly diabetes mellitus, inefficient sugar management resulting in excess body sugar.

E-100: Food coloring agent as a yellow pigment.

Enterocolitis: Inflammation of the digestive tract, involving enteritis of the small intestine and the colon.

Enzyme: A substance produced by living organism that acts as a catalyst to bring about a specific biochemical reaction.

Epidermis: The outer layer of cells on the human skin.

Epilepsy: Any one of a group of disorders of brain function characterized by recurrent sudden attacks.

Essential oils: A volatile oil derived from an aromatic plant constituting the odorous principles of a plant.

Ethereal: Extremely delicate, graceful, elegant, dainty, exquisite and light in a way that seems too perfect for this world.

Exfoliator: (cosmetology). A cosmetic technique that aims to remove dead skin from the body and face.

Exhaustion: A state of extreme physical or mental fatigue.

Fatigue: Extreme tiredness, typically resulting from mental or physical exertion or illness.

Fetus: Is an animal's prenatal stage between the embryonic stage and birth.

Food coloring: Synthetic food dyes, many of which have been linked with tumors in animal studies.

Freckles: A small patch of light brown color on the skin, often becoming more pronounced through exposure to the sun.

Fungus: is any member of the group of eukaryotic organisms that includes microorganisms such as yeasts and molds, as well as the more familiar mushrooms.

Furunculus: A localized pyogenic infection.

Gastritis: Inflammation in a stomach lining.

Gelatin: Is an animal protein mixture.

Genitalia: A sex organ.

Gout: is a form of inflammatory arthritis characterized by recurrent attacks of a red, tender, hot and swollen joint.

Halitosis: Technical term for a bad breath.

Hemisphere: A half of a sphere. A half of the Earth.

Hemoglobin: A red protein responsible for transporting oxygen in the blood of vertebrates.

Hemorrhoids: Enlargement of the normal spongy blood-filled vessels in the wall of the anus.

High-fructose corn syrup: (HFCS). Is a common sweetener in sodas and fruit flavored drinks made from corn starch.

Hoarse: A persons voice sounding rough, typically as the result of a sore throat or of shouting.

H-pylori: Bacteria that infect the lining of the stomach.

Hypertension: High blood pressure.

IBS: Irritable Bowel Syndrome.

Immune system: The body's protective system which provides antibodies to defend against infection and diseases.

Influenza: Is a viral infection that attacks respiratory systems, commonly known as the flu.

Insomnia: Difficulty falling asleep.
Iodine: A trace element necessary to thyroid gland function.

Lactose: A sugar present in milk.
Laxative: Substances that loosen stools and increase bowel movements.
Lubricate: Apply a substance such as oil or grease to the skin to minimize friction and allow smooth movement.

Malignancy: A term for diseases with the presence of a malignant tumor, cancer.
Microbes: A microorganism, especially a bacterium causing disease.
Metabolism: The chemical processes that occur within a living organism in order to maintain life.

Neuralgia: A stabbing pain along a nerve pathway.
Nitrates and nitrites: Frequently added to processed meats as preservatives

Osteoarthritis: Is a type of joint disease that results from breakdown of joint cartilage and underlying bone.
Osteoporosis: Is a bones disease that occurs when the bones losses too many minerals, resulting in their becoming brittle and liable to fracture.
Ovaries: The part of the female reproductive system that produces eggs and female hormones.

Parkinson: Is a progressive nervous system disorder that effects movement,
Periodontitis: Is an inflammatory bacterial disease of the periodontium. It is the most common cause of tooth loss in adults.
Pectin: A soluble gelatinous polysaccharide that is present in ripe fruits and is extracted for use as a setting agent in jams and jellies.
Pharyngitis: Is inflammation of the back of the throat. It typically results in a sore throat and fever.
Psoriasis: Is a chronic skin condition that can cause red, scaly patches of skin to appear.
Psyllium: Is a form of fiber made from the husks of the Plantago ovata seeds. Psyllium is able to pass through digestive system without being completely broken down.
Puja: For the Hindu devotee is making a spiritual connection with the divine.

Rachitis: Old fashioned medical term for rickets. Is an inflammatory affliction of young, growing bones and mostly involves the ribs and long bones of the legs. Caused by lack of Vitamin D

Scurvy: Is a disease resulting from a lack of vitamin C
Seizure: Is a sudden uncontrolled electrical disturbance in the brain.
Sinusitis: Inflammation of one or more sinuses in the facial bones that communicate with the nose, caused by infection or allergic response.
Spondylitis: Is an arthritic inflammation of the vertebra
Stomatitis: Inflammation of the mouth and lips
Sucralose: Is a zero-caloric artificial sweetener.

Thrombophlebitis: Inflammation of the wall of a vein.
Trans-fats: Increasing the risk of heart attack and stroke.
Tuberculosis: (TB). Is an infection disease usually causes by the bacterium Mycobacterium tuberculosis. Generally effects lungs, but can affect other parts of the body.

Ulcers colitis: Is an inflammatory bowel disease that effects the inner most lining of large intestine (colon) and rectum.

Yunani medicine: Is a term for Perso-Arabic traditional medicine practiced in Mughal India and in Muslim cultures in South and Central Asia.

Appendix One: Measurement and Conversion Charts

US Dry Volume Measurements

MEASURE	EQUIVALENT
1/16 teaspoon	dash
⅛ teaspoon	a pinch
3 teaspoon	1 tablespoon
⅛ cup	2 tablespoons (= 1 standard coffee scoop)
¼ cup	4 tablespoon
⅓ cup	5 tablespoons plus 1 teaspoon
½ cup	8 tablespoons
¾ cup	12 tablespoons
1 cup	16 tablespoons
1 pound	16 ounces

US liquid volume measurements

1 quart	2 pints (=4 cups)
1 gallon	4 quarts (=16 cups)

US to Metric Conversions

⅕ teaspoon	1 ml (ml stands for milliliter, one thousandth of a liter)
1 teaspoon	5 ml
1 tablespoon	15 ml
1 fluid oz.	30 ml
⅕ cup	50 ml
1 cup	240 ml
2 cups	470 ml
4 cups	0.95 liters
1 gallon	3.8 liters
1 oz.	28 grams
1 pound	454 grams

Metric to US Conversions

1 milliliter	⅕ teaspoon
5 ml	1 teaspoon
15 ml	1 tablespoon
30 ml	1 fluid oz.
100 ml	3.4 fluid oz.
240 ml	1 cup
1 liter	34 fluid oz.
1 liter	4.2 cups
1 liter	2.1 pints
1 liter	1.06 quarts

1 liter	0.26 gallon
1 gram	0.035 ounce
100 grams	3.5 ounces
500 grams	1.10 pounds
1 kilogram	2.205 pounds
1 kilogram	3.5 oz.

Oven Temperature Conversions

Fahrenheit	Celsius
275 F	140 C
300 F	150 C
325 F	165 C
350 F	180 C
375 F	190 C
400 F	200 C
425 F	220 C
450 F	230 C
475 F	250 C

Ratios for selected foods

Measure	Equivalents

Butter

1 Tbsp (½ oz)	14 grams
1 tablespoon	1/8 cup
1 stick 4 oz	113 grams
8 tablespoons	1 cup
4 sticks (16 oz)	452 grams
32 tablespoons	2 cups

Lemon

1 lemon	1 to 3 tablespoons juice	1 to 1½ tbsp zest
4 large lemons	1 cup juice	¼ cup grated zest

Chocolate

1 ounce	¼ cup grated	40 grams
6 ounces	chips 1 cup chips	160 grams
Cocoa powder	1 cup	115 grams

FOOD RECIPES and PREPARATIONS

Kugel (potato dish) with turmeric 35
Lemon, ginger and mint drink 116
Lemon and honey drink 116
Magic neek soup 91
Pancakes made from æarmers cheese and flour with carrots 97
Persimmon salad with apples and pomegranates 108
Pkhali a snack with spinach and nuts 73
Romantic evening 31
  hot chocolate for two persons 31
Salad with apple cider vinegar 160
Stewed sauerkraut 65
Sweet potatoes with apples and cinnamon 82
Tabouli couscous salad 137
Tomato salad with goat cheese 76
Walnuts for breakfast 118
Zucchini pancakes 80

Plant Name and Other Important Subjects Index

Bold type indicates plant warning, other side effects.

Important Subject Index

Subject Index

duct stones 33

E
e-coli 51
eczema 19, 33, 44, 170
eggplant 183
elixir of health 45, 192
elixir of youth 201
energy boosters 13, 122, 151, 156, 200
enterocolitis 149
epidermis 29
epilepsy 118
erosion 101
essential oils 177, 204
eye 51, 53
    bath 179
    cream 170
    dark circles 179
    epithelial layers 128
    ethereal beauty 38
    lashes 172
    pressure 51
    puffy and tired 186
    swollen 185, 186
exfoliator 209
exhaustion 72, 77

F
face 43
    cleansers 170, 204
    masks 57, 79, 96, 171, 204, 205, 206
    moisturizing and hydrating 43, 174, 204, 205
    nourisher 43
    scrubs 170, 214
    soften: preparation 96
    toner 159
farmer's cheese 148
    preparation 148
fatigue 20, 93, 114, 115, 189
fetus 210
fever 154, 156
fibers 51, 136, 140
figure 195
flexibility 173
flu 26, 85, 93, 114, 117, 155, 156, 180
food 163, 164, 193

oats 164
obesity 15, 16, 149, 210
odors 216
oils 169, 170, 171, 172, 173, 174, 175, 176, 178
    body calming 177
    massage 173
    moisturizers 170, 172, 174, 175 176
    preparation 169, 170, 173
ointment 43, 173
omega-3 28, 64, 67, 118, 133
omega-6 28, 67
omega-9 173
onion peals 88, 89
    Ester eggs 89
osteoarthritis 105
osteochondrosis 201
osteoporosis 68, 120, 133, 144, 146, 149, 155, 159, 182
ovaries 129
overheated fats 192
overweight 159

P
pancreas 38, 51, 112, 128, 149
pancreatic diseases 149
pancreatitis 33
paranoia 47
paralysis 103, 173
parasites 93, 115
Parkinson 20, 47, 153, 154
parodontitis 37, 201
pharyngitis 201
physical capacity 79
peppercorns 163
perfume 25, 178
pigmentary stains 44, 93, 106, 189, 190
pigment 32
pine cones 184
posture 143
potassium 29, 43, 51, 81, 95, 105, 120, 121, 124
pregnancy 33, 47, 72, 133, 175
    pigmentary stains 189
    precautions 47
    skin sensitive 45
    strengthen the muscles 103
    stretch marks 176
probiotics 146

prostheses 214
psoriasis 95, 98, 121, 170, 174
psychiatric syndromes 47
psyllium 44
puja 32

Q
quinoa 140, 164

R
rachitis 115
radiation 133
radioactive isotopes 77, 134
rashes 38, 51
rectal cancer 147
reflux 187
religious rituals 25, 46
repellents 213
reproductive health in men 118
respiratory 16, 61, 68, 72, 103, 155, 180, 195
reumatism 51, 53, 60, 70, 173, 185, 200

S
saccharin 167
saliva 28
scalp treatment 85, 173, 174, 175, 176
scars 44
scented candles 210
sclerosis 88
scrubs 38
scurvy 52, 180
sea cabbage 197
seborrhea 106
seizures 47
selenium toxicity 121
shampoo 210, 215
shaving cream 171
shoes sore 172
shower gel 210
sinus nodules 173
sinusitis 173, 191
    preparation 192
skin 29, 33, 39, 41, 43, 59, 69, 72, 75, 77, 79, 92, 99, 203
    acidity 38, 108
    bath 215
    cleaning: preparation 39

Bibliography

Hildegard von Bingen's, **Medicine, Folk Wisdom Series**, by Dr. Wighard Strehlow (Autor), Gottfried Hertzka MD (Autor), Bear and Company, Inc 1988.

By Hildegard, Hildegard Bingen, Mary Palmquist, John S. Kulas Patric Madigan, **Holistic Healing**, St. Benedict Inc. Collegeville, Minnesota 1994.

John F Nunn, **Ancient Egyptian Medicine**, London 1996.

Andrew Chevallier, **Encyclopedia of Herbal Medicine**, DK Publishing Inc.1996.

Nick Brownlee, **This is Cannabis**, Sanctuary, Publishing Ltd London 2002.

Ona Ragauskiene, Silvija Rimkiene, Valdas Sasnauskas, **Encyclopedia of Medicinal Plants**, Lutute, Kaunas, Lithuania 2005.

Juozas Vasiliauskas, **Plants and Health**, Mokslas, Lithuania 1991.

Juozas Vasiliauskas, **Natural Pharmacy**, Litera Vilnius, Lithuania 2010.

Victor H. Mair, Erling Hoh, **The True History of Tea**, Mintis, Lithuania 2011.

Andrius Rebzdys, **1000 Tips of Healthy Nutrition, What Kind of Food is Medicine**, Dajalita, Lithuania 2013

Maja F Gogulan, **Ideal Health. Food that Heals**, Obuolys, Lithuania 2010.

Katsuzo Nishi, **System of Health Engineering**, Kessinger Publishing 2003.

Padma Lakshmi, **The Encyclopedia of Spices and Herbs**, Ecco 2016.

Peter Wohlleben, **Mysterious Tree Life**, Kitos Knygos, Lithuania, 2018.

Mohring Wolfgang, **Healthy Tea Book, (Best Herbal Mix Recipes)**, Tyrai, Lithuania 2000.

Ilze Jansone, **Trees in Medical Treatment and practical magic**, Ilze Jansone, Lithuania 2016.

Ilze Jansone, **Nature is Healing, Nature is Feeding**, Ilze Jansone, Lithuania 2012.

Ilze Jansone, **1000 Folk Medicine Advice**, Ilze Jansone, Lithuania 2006.

Hannelore Mezei, **Health and Beauty**, Avicena, Lithuania 1998.

Author's Team, **Plants and Cosmetic**, Mokslas, Lithuania 1987.

Jana Tomashkova, **Caring of the Health and Beauty**, Vilnius, Lithuania 1963.

Nijole Degutiene, **Beautiful, Healthy and Strong Hair, Hair Care Oils**, Published White Ark, Lithuania 2014.

Norman W Walker, **Water Can Undermine Your Health**, Canada 1974.

Michal Tombak, **How to Live Long and Healthy Life**, Asveja, Lithuania 2005.

Robin Murphy, **Simple Help From Many Troubles, www.vlmedicina.lt** 2011.

Johhana Budwig, **The Day in the Budwig Diet**, UEsher Production 2011.

Maire Suitsu, Pille Enden, **Holiday dishes with gelatin**, Laisvos valandos, Lithuania 2011.

Leonidas Skliarevskis, **Nutrition Healing Properties and Plants**, Vyriausioji enciklopediju redakcija, Lithuania 1985.

Juozas Ruolia, **Health**, Vilnius, Lithuania 2013.

Author's Team, **Medicinal Plants**, Mintis, Lithuania 1973.

Kurt Schnaubelto, **New Aromatherapy**, Kvapu namai, Lithuania 2012.

P J Pierson Mary Shipley, **Aromatherapy for Everyone**, Square One Publishers 2004.

Sarah Turner, **Garden. Ecology. Health**, Vilnius, Lithuania 2013.

Julia Andrejeva, **Healing Oils**, Satwa, Lithuania 2013.

Laura B Mc, **Bridge Cooking with Ancient Grains**, Create Space Independent Publishing Platform 2013.

Internet

Tissue Repair, Paranormal.lt 07/15/2016.

Grassland, herbs, folk medicine, Paranormal.lt 2017.

Safest to use household cleaning products 2011, 2014, 2015, 2018.

This is exactly what happens when are drinking a can of Coke 2015.

12 ways to use a vinegar 2014, 2016.

15 toxic household products you should stop buying. 2018.

Silent killers in your home 2010, 2014, 2016, 2018.

Newspapers

Journal Sentinel. Cold crushed tea. Published Milwaukee WI 2017.

Magazines

Weekly World News, Canada, Honey and Cinnamon, Published 1995.

Week Savory food and good medicine, Published 2008, 2018.

AARP The sweet'n lowdown, Published 1958-2008.

AARP By Jessica Levine, Eat clean get lean, Published 2015.

Bulletin

AARP Healing foods, Published March and April 2006.

AARP What worse than sugar?, Published 2004.

AARP Live longer, Published 2006, 2017.

www.ingramcontent.com/pod-product-compliance
Lightning Source LLC
Chambersburg PA
CBHW041419290326
41932CB00042B/16